The Nurse Who Became a Rock Star
By Rick Long

Text copyright © 2013 H. Richard Long

All Rights Reserved

ISBN: 9781520699592

Dedication

To God in Heaven.

May God shine down on your life a light as bright as the one shined down upon me. May you realize the presence of that light in your life faster than I did.

If you are facing cancer, maybe I can help you with some tips and tricks that I developed during my cancer journey. It is my prayer that this book will help you find your way through the maze that lies between diagnosis and new life.

Warning: This book mentions God and prayer. If you have cancer, or care about someone who does, you will come to rely on both.

Note: A list of my tips and tricks for surviving cancer, useful for quick referencing, can be found in the Appendix.

Table of Contents

Dedication 3

Foreword 6

Chapter One: It Begins With Diagnosis 8

Chapter Two: What's Wrong With Me? 22

Chapter Three: What is Cancer? 29

Chapter Four: The Workup for Surgery 35

Chapter Five: Surgery 45

Chapter Six: Radiation 56

Chapter Seven: Chemotherapy 66

Chapter Eight: Dark Days 71

Chapter Nine: Christmas and Cancer 75

Chapter Ten: Recovery Phase: I Am Alive! .. 81

Chapter Eleven: The Road to Recovery 88

Chapter Twelve: Chemo Brain 92

Chapter Thirteen: I Don't Do Broken 95

Chapter Fourteen: Return to Nursing. 98

Chapter Fifteen: Who is Victoria and Why Would Someone Want to Kill Her? 100

Chapter Sixteen: Welcome to Iowa 106

Chapter Seventeen: Welcome to Arkansas .. 111

Table of Contents

**Chapter Eighteen: You CAN Go Back
Home Again** 116

**Chapter Nineteen: The Nurse Becomes a
Rock Star** 119

Chapter Twenty: Oh, But God's Not Done.....126

Chapter Twenty-One: We Are All Rock Stars 131

Epilogue: Five Years Out and Counting 133

**Appendix: Nurse Rick's Tips and Tricks for
Surviving Head and Neck Cancer** 134

Foreword

I was a nurse. I had cancer. Now I'm a rock star.

Three simple sentences; a mere twelve words. How funny that such few words can represent so much time and effort, so much pain and sorrow, and eventually so much joy and delight.

They represent a journey really. A business trip of sort. Fate books your flight, sets the meeting agenda, and assigns tasks to be completed. The problem is, Fate seems to have no consideration for your desires, passions, readiness, or level of faith. But if you pay attention, you will find that Fate really does have those areas in mind and is trying to help you grow in each one.

Life, at some point or another, is going to slap you in the face just to get your attention. This has happened to me more than once. At no time in life is this more true than when you find out that you have cancer.

First and foremost, if you have been diagnosed with cancer you are about to go through an experience that will change your life and yet save your life at the same time. It will not be easy but it will not be that hard considering the alternative.

A cousin in Texas had breast cancer a few years ago. She gave me several pieces of advice when I was first diagnosed. Three stand out in my mind still today.

Number one, when you have cancer you find out who your friends are. Some will surprise you. Some will disappoint you. Keep the true friends and let the others go.

Second, nausea is a hydration problem. Whenever she was nauseated during treatments, increasing her fluid intake usually took care of the problem. I found that to be quite true for myself as well.

Thirdly, she told me that I would be a different person when this was all over. She advised that I begin early to decide who that person was going to be. I did and it made all the difference. I decided I was going to be a survivor. I made up my mind that I would live. There was never any doubt that some things would change nor that it was time for some things to change. And never any question that I would have to be, with God's help, the one to change them.

Fate slapped me in the face with cancer. This time, I slapped back. It was not easy.

Chapter One: It Begins With Diagnosis

"Take a deep breath. Hold it in." The CAT Scan machine makes a whirring sound as the table I'm lying on suddenly moves forward. The tech running the machine from the next room comes back on the speaker, "OK Mr. Long, let it out. Now let's do that again. Deep breath. Hold it."

Again, the machine moves my head and neck through a swirling x-ray pattern that will produce pictures of the inside of my body. The radiologist and I are on a hunt. The doctors I've seen recently know something is in there. We can feel the evidence. We can put our fingers on the lump in my neck. We can poke it with a needle and take a sample of fluid from it. Funny how reaching up to scratch your beard one Sunday night while driving home, and feeling a bump the size of a small egg in your neck, can change the rest of your life.

Right now, our job is to come up with an opinion on what the lump might be. Darnedest thing though; I already know what it is. I knew it the minute I felt it. It is throat cancer. Funny that thousands of dollars will be spent trying to prove what I already know to be true. Couldn't we just bypass all this expense, and pain, and start trying to get it out of there?

I know it is not that simple. We have to

determine if the cancer is malignant or benign. Fancy words, eh? I call medical terms such as those, "ten dollar words" because the more of those words the doctor uses, the higher your bill is going to be.

Malignant means the cancer can, and probably already has, spread to other places in your body. Benign means it will just make a mess where it is. The fluid I talked about, or maybe a tissue sample, is sent to a lab where people smarter than me about such things will look it over and proclaim what they think it is. I'll want to think they are wrong at first but most of the time they aren't. They wouldn't have a job if they were wrong the first time out on every case now would they? Sadly, no.

This is not a process that I am unfamiliar with. The problem this time is I'm on the wrong side of the equation. For the past 23 years, I've been a Registered Nurse. I have taken countless patients through this process. I watch the CAT scan from the control booth then transport the patient back to their hospital room. Next I help them understand the results because when the doctor rushes into the patient's room for five minutes the next morning, he or she won't wait for the light of understanding to go on in the patient's eyes before heading off to the next patient. Not all doctors are like that but some are. Too many, for sure.

So me, Nurse Rick, follows the doctor and re-explains the results, the implications, and the next step in the plan. What I'm really doing is instilling hope. If the patient has hope that things will get better, there is a chance that they will. If the patient loses hope that things will ever be better, that's a very dangerous mindset. I don't know the secret that triggers death but it is not far from there, wherever it is, whatever it is.

As I lay on the scanner table, I think to myself what an odd profession nursing really is. If I told you I worked in construction, you would instantly have in mind some concept of what I do for a living. You would take the vision of me you could see, the six foot, one inch frame, the neatly tied pony tail, the dark eyes, and tan skin and you would put me in a scene inside the bare framework of a house going up with a hammer in my hand or maybe laying brick or running around with a wheel barrow filled with something or other. Blue-collar work, they call it. I could do that. You would know what that is.

I grew up on a farm in the rural south and started driving a tractor when I was in my early teen years. You can envision that. The tan straw hat pulled low on my head with sweat pouring down my face. Dad drives up alongside in his pickup truck in the mid-afternoon to check on me and bring a cold soda. We drive home at dusk for supper with the family. Not outside the realm of what people think of when they imagine what a farm boy does in a day.

I also play the drums. My mom would find me

at age three on the kitchen floor dragging pots and pans out of the lower kitchen cabinets and banging on them with wooden spoons. She was the one who would take me to the local hardware store at age eight to get cardboard boxes so I could build my first drum set, using Tinkertoys® for the stands and metal pieces out of an erector set for cymbals. She's the one that would help load the car with drum cases when I was a teenager and head off to Little Rock for the State Fair Talent Show or to Memphis for the Mid-South Talent Contest. She's the one who would talk Dad into letting me play public gigs at the local dance hall, outside the sanctuary of the church and its safe and sane audience. She is the one who could convince him to spend hard-earned money on a professional drum kit to replace the small Sears kit I started out on. She was my music advocate, my supporter in times of doubt, and always my biggest fan.

She died when I was 17 years old.

You can imagine what a drummer does. Setting up the kit, playing four-hour gigs in a smoke-filled club or an hour and a half on a concert stage, then tearing down the kit, hauling it home, and hoping you get to play again soon. You can imagine a family torn apart by the death of a central figure, the jealousies when Dad moves on to a second wife with two children of her own, and the loneliness of a young serviceman thousands of miles from home who joined up just for the slim hope of getting a ticket to California where his music career could have some chance of success. Then after earning a degree in music with his GI Bill money, he hears the voice of God tell him to go to nursing school so he could have income to support his passion for music and he becomes a Registered Nurse. This is not outside the realm of what you can imagine.

The tech's voice comes over the speaker again. "Mr. Long, we're going to inject the dye now. You'll feel a warm sensation like you're peeing in your pants. Don't worry, you're not really. It just feels like it."

"Great," I think dolefully to myself.

I don't believe most people know what nurses really do. The public vision of nursing involves images from sitcom television shows where handsome men and cutesy women sit around flirting with one another all day until they have to deal with minor interruptions from the patients. Sure, some of that goes on. Not much, though. What nurses really do is something entirely different.

Here's how my typical day as a nurse starts. It's five o'clock in the morning. The phone rings. It's the registry company I work for. You see, I still wanted to be a musician so I did not want to lock myself into a situation where someone else controlled my schedule. Most nurses have to work every other weekend and weekends are about the only time musicians work. Sure, the studio players work during the week but there are not many musicians that make a living that way. Most people who play music do it for little or no pay on weekends in clubs or churches. By signing up with a staffing company, I could choose the days I wanted to work and be free to take whatever music jobs I could find.

On the phone is one of the "staffers," usually a young adult in their 20's, who has been calling all the hospitals in the Inland Empire area of southern California to ask the evening supervisor if more nurses are needed for the day shift. This is the area where I lived, and this is how I worked, for most of my nursing career.

I answer the phone still half asleep. "This is Rick."

"Good morning, Rick. I've got you booked for ICU at Loma Linda today."

"Thanks. Kids or adults?"

"They said they were still deciding."

"OK. I'll be there. Bye."

Loma Linda University Hospital is the local teaching facility. San Bernardino Community Hospital is much smaller but also a good source of work for me. Sometimes neither of those hospitals is busy and I drive out to Palm Springs to work. I've worked every hospital in the area at one time or another. But five o'clock in the morning is when I find out where I'm going for the day.

Now I shower, dress, and drive. Run into Starbucks. Drive a little more. Ride a shuttle bus from the parking lot to the hospital's back door. Follow someone else who is coming to work through the door because registry nurses are not allowed to have a badge that will work the electronic lock. Go to the staffing office. They tell me which of their various intensive care units (ICU) I'm working. I ride the elevator to the unit and find the charge nurse, then receive the number of a room that contains two patients that I will take responsibility for during the next 12 and a half hours.

What is it I do for these patients? Unfortunately, everything. ICU patients are the sickest of the sick. It is as near dead as you can be and still be living on this planet. If they have to go to the bathroom, I have to take them. If they can't walk, I have to figure out how to get it out of them right where they lay. Let me tell you, that isn't always easy and it definitely isn't pretty.

They have to have nutrition too. ICU patients don't eat well. Maybe I have to stick a tube down their nose into their stomach and pour something the consistency of melted milk shake down the tube. Not too much though. They might vomit and inhale the fluid and drown right in front of me. They get just enough that they don't lose more weight and become weaker and never get out of ICU. But those bad outcomes still happen sometimes.

The first thing to understand is that this patient is in ICU because something terrible is wrong with them. Maybe they had a car accident and they are all busted up and infection is streaming throughout their body. Maybe they cut themselves innocently enough around the house and didn't even know they were a Diabetic until the wound didn't heal, became infected, and caused them to go what's called "septic" and now they are about to die a horrible death. Or maybe they aren't infected at all and they are here for heart problems, kidney problems, a spontaneous bleeding inside the brain commonly called a "stroke," or some other calamity that has befallen them.

The really sick part is that most nurses will tell you that the more outlandish cases are the interesting ones. After several years of working at the bedside, you have seen it all and to have something unusual going on with a patient can make for a more exciting day.

I don't relish these cases like some nurses do. I'll take the boring ones anytime, thank you. Why? Not because I'm lazy, no sir. I'm the hardest working nurse you will ever see. I'll work four 12-hour shifts a week even though three shifts is considered by all hospitals to be full-time. I'll work different units or at different hospitals if I need to; anything to keep working. I've worked nine shifts in a row trying to get some special days off without losing any pay. Nobody works harder than I do. Nobody.

I like the typical cases because they can be helped. And that's my job.

The one part of nursing people might have a correct vision about is the medications. Tons of meds are given in a day. Intravenous (IV) fluids, IV antibiotics, IV medications, medications by mouth, some by rectum, and some shot right into a muscle with a big needle. The credo of all nurses is "The right medication given to the right patient by the right route in the right amount at the right time for the right reason and documented the right way." For all the rules and regulations that the government puts on the health care system, if we would just follow that one simple statement things would be alright most of the time.

Like the waitresses at your favorite restaurant have an ongoing battle with the cooks, we nurses have a long-standing feud with the hospital's pharmacy. It is not pretty. They think we are incompetent and we think they are inefficient. You see, we can't give any medication unless it comes to us through the pharmacy system.

Once a doctor writes an order for a medication, the pharmacy has to process that order before the medication can be released for the patient. In recent years, machines have been installed on most hospital units that can dispense some of the safer medications. These include acetaminophen, stool softeners, a few pain medications, and maybe a few special medications used often on that unit. You have an identification code and password that allows you into the machine and each med is taken out in the patient's name, recorded by the system, and filed with the pharmacy. The system even alerts the pharmacy when supplies are running low and a pharmacy tech is dispatched to refill the machine. This sounds really great, doesn't it?

It is, for the most part, but often the medication I need for my patient isn't in there. So I have to wait for the supply person to make their hourly rounds with the new meds or I have to go the pharmacy and retrieve it myself. I don't mind walking to the pharmacy except that this is ICU. My patients are never to be left alone for fear they may start to die and no one notice in time to save them. Sometimes we have an extra person on the unit that acts as a "runner" and can help get things from central supply and the pharmacy. Nurses are expensive so managers don't like to schedule extra help. Most of the time, the runner is waiting for a post-op heart transplant or some other extreme case and won't be available to help past the arrival of that patient. So I wait for the med. The patient waits for the med. We all have to wait sometimes.

I'm waiting now myself. I'm waiting for this CAT scan of my neck to be over. While you are lying on your back, staring at the ceiling of the examination room, you can choose to think about what the tumor might look like on the film. You can imagine its size and shape, its consistency, and other aspects. I think instead about my latest motorcycle ride: north on the I-15 up the Cajon Pass from San Bernardino to Victorville after work a couple of nights ago just to get good barbeque.

There's something about riding a motorcycle forty or fifty miles that makes food taste better.

"Mr. Long, hold still. We're going to have to run that one more time." I can see the tech through the glass and he has a serious look on his face. Laughing and joking during a test is not professional behavior. How I wish he was doing that now.

Over the years, I've had to come up with something to help me cope with the stresses of being a nurse. I suppose I'd be a rock star drummer if I could but it seems all of those jobs are taken. It's not all it's cracked up to be anyway. I've met several professional drummers through my side job as a freelance writer for a magazine called "Modern Drummer." The pro drummers tell me what I do as a nurse is more important. I console myself by remembering that statement whenever I'm cleaning a patient's behind while listening to one of them play on Good Morning America or some other television program on the hospital room television.

So music hasn't been my refuge; at least not yet. Something else came along: travel. I suppose I am a bit like a dog in that if you open the car door and say, "Come on, boy, let's go," I'll jump in and around the bend we go. I like seeing different walls. I like the outdoors. I like the feel of the wind in my face. Motorcycle riding takes care of all these little issues quite nicely. I own two Harley-Davidson Sportster models, one of which has a sidecar attached so I can carry more stuff for camping or long trips. The other is dressed in racing colors and fancy decals. I don't race it any more so than any other freeway driver races but it looks fast and makes me excited every time I look at it.

I like thinking of long motorcycle trips, like the annual Yuma, Arizona, run or heading up to Big Sur along the Pacific Coast Highway. I make a lot of those types of rides. For now, I am still lying on the CAT scan table, I wonder what the next ride will be, short or long, and how far off it might be. Should it be some grandiose, marathon adventure? Should it be to the Post Office to get the mail? Will I be able to choose or barely able to do either?

"That's it Mr. Long. We're done. The nurse will take out your IV and you can get dressed."

One of my favorite sayings in life is, "More will be revealed." It acknowledges that we can't know everything that's going to happen and that we have to wait sometimes for more pieces of the puzzle to come into view. This is one of the more aggravating things about our existence but one that must be fully accepted. There is no real alternative. Patience truly is a virtue.

It takes a lot of patience to wait for results from medical testing. The problem is that you know that somebody somewhere in the system has the results you need prior to the information reaching you. Sometimes they may have it days before you get it. In decades past, a biopsy sent to a far away lab would be finished and the result sent to your doctor via a letter in the mail. He or she might not read the letter for a day or so, and then you wouldn't get the news until your appointment next Thursday. Unfair, it seems, that all those people know so much about you so early in the process while you remain in the dark, so to speak, for so long.

In more modern times, the far away lab e-mails the results right to your electronic chart which sends an alert to the ordering physician upon his next log-in to the system. He quickly reads the findings and clicks on your contact info. He grabs the office portable phone and calls your cell phone number. He finds me at work, two minutes before assisting a physician with a tricky intravenous line placement on my patient. He talks to me using words like "cancer" and "malignancy," then tries to comfort me with phrases like, "I know this must come as a shock to you," and "The lymph nodes we tested aren't the primary site and I don't know where it is for sure."

Maybe the old way wasn't so bad. The world turned a little slower in those days. I keep the Thursday appointment and arrive with a list of questions for the doctor. All of them surround the concept of "What's next?"

The answer is that there are a lot of possibilities and few certainties. More tests? That's certain. Surgery? At least one. That's certain. After that, "More will be revealed." The words "radiation" and "chemotherapy" roll off the doctor's tongue so smoothly considering the trouble they actually represent.

I suppose I do that too when I talk to patients. I act calm and serious even though the words are dark and ominous. What would be better? Probably nothing. Health problems are quite scary since much of the time you don't have any control over the outcome. You follow the instructions of someone you barely know, take magic potions concocted by yet another unknown person, and wait. Wait to get better while you rest, hope, pray, and heal. Like I said earlier, we all have to wait sometimes.

Now I'm the patient instead of the nurse. There is not time for a motorcycle trip before the surgery and I will be too weak to take one for months afterward. I have not played a gig on the drums in quite some time but this is one of those moments that being a rock star drummer sure sounds good. Somehow, I know that life is not over yet because I understand from deep inside my soul that I am supposed to spend at least part of this life being a full-time musician or writer. That has not happened yet. Faith that it will is about to be the only thing keeping me alive.

Chapter Two: What's Wrong With Me?

People can sense when something is wrong with you. The ones that care about you will ask and want to know. Others will ask but they do not really want to know.

"What's wrong Rick? You don't seem like yourself today," someone asked at work.

I am still me but something is wrong with me. Is it enough to just say, "I found out I have cancer" and walk away? Will they think that is enough to know too? They do not want to know I am in a bad marriage that went terribly wrong ten years ago and got worse this year. They do not want to know I am up to my eyeballs in debt trying to buy my way into a happier state of mind. They do not want to know I am so burned out with bedside nursing that I dread waking up every day and hate coming to work. They do not want to know and I do not want to think about it.

"Who's your doctor?" is usually the next question they ask.

"Kaiser," I reply and they know just what I mean.

My insurance is with Kaiser, the world's largest Health Maintenance Organization (HMO). It is a massive system with hospitals, clinics, and doctors.

Tons of doctors. None of which I know very well. Oh, I see my primary physician often enough that I kind of know him but we don't have Saturday afternoon barbeques together. It is not like when I was a child in a small rural community and we went to church with the family doctor. Dad doesn't know this guy from the Lodge. He doesn't live one block over from me with a clinic behind his house. No. This is the big city. Cold. Impersonal. Efficient. But it works.

Some of my nursing friends tell me it works because I know "the system." I don't doubt that this is partially true. You see, the patient has to be his or her own best advocate. Yes, the poster on the wall at your clinic or hospital says that there is a "patient advocate" that you can call if you have a problem or just want to gripe about something that happened that you don't like. That's not what I mean. I mean you have to push things along in the system and push like there is no tomorrow. If you do not push, there might not be a tomorrow. Here's an example.

After I felt the lump, I said to myself, "I'm a nurse. I know this might not be just a swollen lymph node. I better have this seen about now." This is in stark difference to how most men handle health problems.

Most men will say, "I don't have to go to the doctor. I'll feel better in a day or two. Hey, I'll go if it falls off" (and we all know what he's talking about falling off. God knows if it did start to fall off he wouldn't hesitate about going to the doctor then!) But I went the very next day. Urgent Care they call it. No appointment necessary. Just show up, get in a long line, try not to breath the spray off the sneeze of the two-year-old with red eyes and a snotty nose next to you, and they'll get to you as soon as they can.

An hour rolls by. I get called into the clinic and the most basic of health care interventions are done: temperature, pulse, respiratory rate, and blood pressure. All are fine, the nurse's aide says. But I know deep inside that I'm not fine. Something is terribly wrong.

The doctor listens to my story about finding the swollen lymph node. He knows I'm a nurse because I told him so. Sometimes medical personnel will believe you better if you let them know that you are "in the business." Sometimes the doctors believe you less because they think you are trying to impress them and they know since they are the top of the food chain in the medical ocean that you couldn't possibly self-diagnose or treat anything serious. They think you are just making their job harder by wasting their time with your cockamamie story and whimsical diagnosis and treatment plan. This happened to a friend who complained of a broken wrist for a year before a doctor finally stopped ordering more x-rays and ordered the more extensive Magnetic Resonance Imaging (MRI) and found the hidden crack. Her surgery to set the wrist would surely have been easier had the break been found shortly after the injury.

The doctor listens and then utters his command: "Go home, take these antibiotics for ten days, and cross your fingers." This doesn't sound promising. He senses something could be wrong too but of course, he must follow the HMO protocol and try the cheap antibiotic "road map" first before ordering an expensive workup.

I do as he says. No other choice is present at this time. I could choose not to do anything but that will not take me to the next level in the HMO treatment game.

On day seven of the antibiotics, the lump in my neck hasn't changed. I make a "same day" appointment with my primary physician and tell him the story. He's a great doctor but not a head/neck specialist so he refers me to another clinic for further diagnostics. That's fancy language for, "I don't know what's wrong with you, I don't know how to figure out for sure what's wrong with you, and I don't want to be the one who treats what's wrong with you, especially if I get it wrong." What's wrong with that?

Nothing I suppose now that the computer is taking over the medical system. When I first started nursing, a referral to another doctor could take weeks. A hand written note or form was mailed to a distant clinic. Someone there would read the consult order, issue an appointment, and send a letter to the patient with the time and date when they would be seen by the specialist. Meanwhile, what's wrong with you isn't getting any better. If anything, it is getting worse. Much worse.

Now the computer has taken the lag time out of the system. My primary doc clicks a box on the consult screen and away the order goes via super-fast broadband digital cabling to the inbox of the head/neck clinic. I was able to take a canceled appointment and get in two days later. We looked inside my sinuses and throat with a camera, and we biopsied the problem lymph node with a syringe and big needle. The doctors and nurses were prompt, thorough, and nice enough.

"Let's get a CAT scan while we're waiting for the biopsy results," the doc suggests.

"Sure," I reply. After all, I'm anxious to get the process started. I already have a strong suspicion of what the biopsy results will be: cancer.

And this is where we started the book. And since this is a book, it needs to be readable. You see, I have been a part-time freelance writer during most of my nursing career. I started writing after a "Letter to the Editor" I wrote and submitted to "The Music and Sound Retailer" magazine led to an offer to write my own column. The publisher also ran "Band and Orchestra Product News" and I soon had a column in that magazine as well. Those were great magazines to write for and I loved the opportunity but my goal was also to get published in "Modern Drummer." I got my foot in the door with them a dozen or more years ago and now I write about drum equipment, events in the drum industry like store openings and such, as well as the occasional interview with some of today's great players. My claim to fame was the assignment to interview Marlon Brando about a device he made for conga drums.

Yes, Marlon Brando was a drummer as well as an actor and invented a better way to manufacture conga drums so that they could be tuned more easily. Amazing. Amazing that I got the assignment! He had not done a magazine article in twenty years but I got the interview, wrote the article, and got to know him a little in the short time left before he passed on.

I told the editors that they had ruined me with that assignment because from now on, even if I was asked to interview the President of the United States I would have to say, "OK fine but it's not like it's Brando or anything." After Brando, whether you are a writer, a television host, a news reporter, or whatever, nothing will ever parallel that experience. He truly was that bright of a star.

There. Now we are not talking about the cancer. Doesn't that feel better? Whew! Makes the book more readable don't you think? The funny thing about having cancer is that you do not think about it all the time. You cannot, really. Life goes on. Someone has to fix meals. Someone has to do laundry. Someone has to drive to the treatment clinic and pay attention to the road. If you are in a bad marriage and live thousands of miles from family, that someone is you.

Oh, I could have asked for help from friends and my wife's local family. They offered. They meant well, really they did. But at the time of the treatments, I lived in a small mountain community with several feet of snow on the ground. The friends and family that offered to help with transportation did not own a four-wheel drive vehicle. They were not coming to my rescue. I had to go out to the truck, dig snow if I had to, put chains on the tires if I had to, do in fact whatever I had to do to get to the treatments just like my life depended upon it. And it did.

Chapter Three: What is Cancer?

Few words strike fear in the hearts of mankind like the word cancer. What is cancer anyway, that it should carry such weight? The answer is quite simple really.

Remember in high school when you studied about the deoxyribonucleic acid found in the nucleus of all cells. No? How about DNA? Yeah, that's the big buzzword now in medicine and law. Take a little of that stuff and we can prosecute you for almost any crime you could commit, prove whether or not you are the parent of a particular child, and maybe even clone you, just to name a few things. It is the core of our cells, the architectural blue print to the design center of our body, the secret stuff to which physical life owes it all. Magic? No. Predictable? Mostly. Fragile? More than you might imagine.

Want to screw up your DNA? It is not that hard. Any number of available street drugs, even the cheapest marijuana, will do it for most guys. It's the sperm that will pay the price first and then of course, the child it produces. Get rid of the drugs, ejaculate the old sperm, then let your body make some new sperm and they'll be fine. The kid will be fine. Unless of course some other genetic malformation occurs.

Yes, women can mess up DNA just as easily as men. Try taking the same street drugs, some prescription drugs, or drink alcohol while you are forming a new life inside you. If it all doesn't kill you it will just about kill the baby. Stop doing those things while the baby is forming and he or she will likely be healthy. If you think life is tough now, try having an unhealthy baby to deal with. That's two lives ruined. Or more if the baby-daddy didn't run off. They'll do that sometimes. They do it a lot when the baby is not healthy.

A late-night comedian might say, "And the number one thing that can go wrong with your DNA is… cancer."

We grow and maintain our bodies through a process called cell division. DNA is the key component for cell division. The DNA divides, reproduces itself, and follows along into the new cell so that whole process can occur over and over again. A true miracle? Yes. It is a miracle that it goes right most of the time.

This cell division thing is a delicate process. If the DNA doesn't reproduce itself just so, the new cell won't be the same as the old cell. That happens for everyone eventually. Take a look at your skin in a picture from your childhood and look at it now. Is it as tight as it was? No? The same color? No? Guess what? The DNA isn't reliably able to reproduce itself correctly forever. It's called "getting old." We age. The more you do to your DNA to screw it up, the faster you age. There's no getting around this fact.

Sometimes, the DNA becomes, let's say, confused. The cell divides and the new cell is nothing like the old cell. There have been cases where surgeons have opened up a lump someone felt and found a tooth. That really doesn't hurt anything other than it is not supposed to be there. It grew for no apparent reason in a place other than the mouth. It's still just a tooth though, or hair, or a piece of bone, or just some bodily tissue that is in a place where it is not usually found. This is a benign tumor. Benign is a buzzword for "this isn't going to hurt anything or spread anywhere else."

But sometimes, the DNA divides and something awful happens. The new cell is not like the old cell but not really like any other cells in the body either. It is growing fast, taking in sugar/glucose faster than any cell around it, and multiplying quickly. It's growing so fast that it can't contain itself and spreads to surrounding tissues and maybe even to the lymph system which is the garbage service for your biological trash.

This is a malignant cancer that will grow until it disturbs the function of nearby nerves or blood vessels, that might spread to major organs and cause them to deteriorate dramatically, and that left untreated, will eventually cause death through any number of ways, all involving the destruction of a major organ like the brain, lungs, liver, and such.

God, fate, nature, or whatever your belief system dictates did a pretty good job of designing the body. Many of the most important internal and external features come in pairs so that if you have something happen to one of them, you have a spare ready to go. Eyes, arms, and legs are a good example of this. We even have ten fingers and ten toes. Somebody must have thought we would loose a lot of those things. And any nurse who has worked in the Emergency Department for any length of time will tell you that in truth, we do.

Inside the body, you will find two lungs and two kidneys. These organs are especially important. You can only live a few moments without oxygen processed by the lungs. You might make a few days without kidneys to filter out the poisons produced by the normal chemical reactions that go on in your body. Yes, life depends upon the major organs for daily survival.

Unfortunately, the designers of the human body were trapped by the same laws of physics that control the rest of the universe. There is only one heart. You cannot easily design a two-pump circulatory system. There is one brain. Two thinking brains in one body? No way. This would be worse than the interpersonal friction that goes on between you and your sibling, spouse, or worst enemy. One brain is all you can have. The digestive tract and urinary tract suffer the same limitations. One each is provided and only one. If malignant cancer gets into one of these single organs, the only alternative is to cut the cancer out, if it isn't too big and you can do it without further damaging the organ, or you can transplant the organ from a human donor.

How many times have I heard someone say, "I'll just keep on doing what I'm doing [usually smoking and/or drinking] and if I need a new organ, I'll get a transplant." How nice it would be if it were that easy. Transplants are a pain for several reasons. First, organs are hard to come by. The tissue has to match your specific tissue type, the organ has to be reasonable close to the size of the old one, and someone has to die most of the time for you to get one. Kidney transplants are about the only organ transplant that can be done without killing the donor body.

By default, if you have an organ transplant, it is a used organ you are getting. And by the way, you know how easy it is to abuse your organs. The person you got the replacement organ from just might have been doing the same thing you were doing or worse. There's no ten-year/100,000 mile warranty with your organ transplant. You get a little borrowed time in life with no guarantee as to how much. Better be thinking about how you are going to use that time. It's definitely running out.

We haven't even talked about the medication that you will have to take forever and ever. The immune system that saves your life from germs and such doesn't much like organs that were originally in someone else. You will have to take medications every day called immunosuppressants that stop the function of the immune system for the rest of your life. How much of this medication will I have to take, you ask? Who knows. You will have to experiment with the dosage to find out what works for you and it varies a lot from person to person.

Frequent hospitalizations, set backs, organ failures, and medication trial and error plague the transplant patient. This is not to say that it can't work for you, but realistically your chances are slim to none that you would even get an organ much less that it would work well once installed. If you get cancer in a major organ, you've really got problems. Fortunately for me, if anything about cancer can be called fortunate, mine turned out to be in a rather small organ: my left tonsil.

Chapter Four: The Workup for Surgery

"I'm taking you to surgery next Tuesday," the surgeon pronounced. "I can look in your throat and try to find the cancer here in the office but I can REALLY look in your throat when you are asleep on the operating table."

"Great," I think to myself.

I'd never had surgery before. Didn't want it, wouldn't want it, and always thought I might even say no if it every came up that I needed it. Yep, typical "guy" response. In my nursing life, I take care of post-op patients all the time. Post-op is one of those fancy medical terms that mean you just came out of surgery. Why can't we just say that? "Nurse Rick, I'm assigning you a patient that just came out of surgery," instead of, "Hey, you're getting a fresh post-op." Almost sounds like a breakfast snack doesn't it?

"Hey Honey, I'm going to the store for more post-ops. Want me to get some bread while I'm there? OK, back in a minute." Life without humor is no life at all.

Going to surgery isn't simple. There are some hoops to jump. First, the HMO lawyer says that the surgeon must determine if the patient is healthy enough for surgery. This is an interesting twist. If I was really healthy, I wouldn't need surgery now would I? So a fine line has to be drawn between being well enough to withstand the surgery needed to make you healthier and sick enough that you shouldn't risk having the surgery and that you might as well accept that you are going to be sick for a long while because they're not fixing you. Is there humor somewhere in that statement? Hmmm.

The heart is the first thing they check. An electrocardiogram or EKG is run to make sure your heart can stand the strain of being cut on, poked at, yanked on and whatever else they do down there in the basement under the lights. Yeah, I know it should be called ECG but for eons it has been referred to as an EKG instead. I do not have a clue why.

My EKG goes well. I know I suffer from occasional atrial fibrillation. I wake up at night and feel like I have a motor running in my chest. It is strong enough that it feels like the washing machine in the laundry room is on spin cycle. Sometimes when I feel this, the washing machine actually is on spin cycle so I have to listen for that first but if it isn't, I just hold my breath deeply for a moment, then breathe out slowly until all my air is out and then hold that condition for a few seconds. This massive movement of the lungs irritates the nearby heart just enough to stimulate it out of the fibrillation. I go back to sleep. No big deal, I tell myself. Again, a typical guy response.

It is a big deal if it doesn't stop. When the top part of your heart vibrates instead of beating in rhythm it doesn't pump out as much blood as it should. If the blood isn't moving enough, it may clot. If it clots and that clot moves out of the heart and into the rest of the body it can plug up the circulatory system. You might even get really unlucky and have a bunch of clots (a shower of clots) move out all at once and lodge in the lungs (pulmonary embolism), or legs (deep vein thrombosis), or the brain (occlusive cerebral vascular accident). There is a group of "ten dollar words" that will get you in trouble.

None of these is good and the one in the brain is the worst of all. You can put your leg up and not walk for a few days while the drug Heparin circulates through your body to break up the clot. The one in your lung is treated basically the same way but once the brain tissue past the roadblock dies, it is dead. Smart medical personnel will tell you that other parts of the brain can take over the function of the dead part but that doesn't happen easily. If I tell you it is going to, it might because you will go to therapy and try to get it to do so. That's the best. If I tell you it won't ever, you won't even try and guess what, it for sure won't ever get better.

So when my little breathing trick doesn't work anymore, then I'll have to go to the emergency room and be admitted to the cardiac unit. I've worked as a registry nurse on that unit at my local Kaiser hospital and the unit is a bit old looking and not too pretty. The nurses are OK and I don't know the docs. I suppose they give good care but it is not a very pleasant atmosphere. I don't want to go there so I'll keep doing the little breathing routine to myself for as long as it works.

The big risk for me is if I go into fibrillation during the surgery. It is not life threatening so to speak. The surgeon will be notified of it right away by the anesthesiologist, scrub nurse, or whoever sees it on the cardiac monitor first. I'll be given drugs or a little electric shock to bring me out of it. Problem is, when the surgery is over, I'll be transferred to that cardiac unit I don't like and labeled a heart patient for the remainder of my life. Oh the trouble that will bring!

"Any heart trouble?" the surgeon asks during the workup interview.

"I did a Holter Monitor one time a few years ago but it didn't find anything." A Holter monitor is a device about the size of a large iPod that has wires that connect to your chest and record your EKG for 24 hours. You have a piece of paper that you write down things on like the times when you are eating, sleeping, exercising, etc., and if you feel chest pain or anything else of an unusual nature. When you take the device back to the clinic where you got it, someone looks over the graph, focusing on the times you put down when something might have been happening.

The surgeon grunts and moves on to the next question. As long as my EKG is good and I deny any obvious heart problems, he's good to go. No sense in looking for more trouble. That's not the HMO way.

The surgeon and/or his nurse ask me more questions about my health. All go by without raising any flags, even the story about what happened in nursing school when I nearly died one morning.

Here is the story. In anatomy lab, you have to learn the muscles and organs of the body. To help you understand musculature, they make you cut open dead cats. It would be better if you could cut open dead people but they are much harder and more expensive to come by than dead cats so they are saved for training doctors and surgeons. Nurses get the cats.

Since dead cats aren't really free either, you have to pick a lab partner and the two of you work on one cat. This brings up another issue that nursing students who are male must contend with: female lab partners.

You see, no matter if the female lab partner is kind, helpful, plain looking with small breasts and a simple hairdo, your wife or girlfriend or significant other thinks that this lab partner is the most threatening beast ever to roam the face of the earth. The wife thinks that the lab partner must have blond bouffant hair, dark eyes, breasts the size of watermelons, and wants to drop her drawers in the elevator on the way out of the building so you can have sex with her right then and there. Let me assure you that in reality, nothing could be farther from the truth. Instead, my lab partner almost killed me.

My lab partner was nice enough to work with, outgoing enough to be helpful, but so inexperienced that while we are cutting on the cat one Friday, she nicked my finger with the scalpel. It wasn't a very big cut. It was nothing that required stitches or anything more than some antibiotic cream and a small bandage. Nothing that would prevent me from spending the weekend at my Dad's farm, riding ATVs and hiking in the nearby woods. Everything was fine until Monday morning.

Back at college to start the week, I awoke to the sound of the alarm clock, sat up on the side of the bed, and immediately experienced the worst headache of my life. I don't get headaches usually. This was a massive one.

I reached for my pants, pulled them up, then looked at my hands. I knew I was supposed to use my hands to pull my pants together and button them but somehow, I could not make my hands move in that way. This went on for some time until my wife came in, saw what was going on, and had me lay back down. She later said that I mentioned seeing my deceased mother that morning in the room.

She called my professor to let him know that I wouldn't be in class that day. At a small college, you get the kind of personal attention that might save your life.

He asked what was wrong with me and she said that I had a headache, seemed confused, and was having trouble moving around. He said for her to call for an ambulance immediately and she did.

Though I vaguely remember being loaded into the ambulance, I don't remember having a lumbar puncture procedure, commonly called a spinal tap, done at the emergency room. If you've ever had one of those or seen one done on someone you care about, you know how unusual it would be not to remember it.

The results of the pressure-reading portion of the test were known immediately. My intracranial pressure was terribly high. Plans were quickly developed to move me to Memphis so a neurosurgeon could take me to the operating room and remove the top of my skull to relieve the pressure before my brain was permanently damaged by the reduced blood flow, a tragic side effect of too much pressure inside the head.

Fortunately, there is also a lab test portion, where fluid from my spinal column, the same fluid that your brain floats in, is tested for infection. Just as they were about to move me , a lab tech came running into the emergency cubicle where I was laying shouting, "We got it. He's got encephalitis."

Now the plan changes instantly. I'm given intravenous steroids to reduce the swelling and antibiotics to combat the infection. I'm moved to a room on the medical floor. I do remember the minister from my church coming by, taking my hand, and praying aloud. Someone had called him and asked him to come by just in case.

I also remember having to go pee. I think I pulled out the IV and crawled out the end of the bed. The bed rails were up so I could not get out the usual way. After peeing all over the bathroom, I simply went back to bed. What the heck, I was tired. It had been a long morning!

The first thing you tell the patient after a lumbar puncture is not to sit up for several hours. This is because your intracranial pressure goes up when you sit up and the small pinhole that was made in your spinal column might reopen and spinal fluid could leak out. This, as you might imagine, is not a desirable event. For one thing, it causes a severe headache, which I already had so now no one can really tell if I have a leaky spine or if I'm still just hurting from the increased pressure problem which, by the way, would really complicate the leaky spine problem if it did develop. So getting up to go to the bathroom was not the best choice. Oh well, I didn't know and no one was watching me. In fact, I never even told anyone about this until just now.

Note to nursing self: patients will hide things from you. Things like not following proper post-procedure protocol or having atrial fibrillation. And they can hide these facts for 30 years or more if they want to. I did.

After I recovered and returned to college, every time I would see the anatomy professor, he called me a "walking miracle." He couldn't believe that after just two weeks recovery time, I was back in school, didn't have any memory or motor function deficits, and could think clearly. He will tell you that I got a mosquito bite on the farm that weekend that carried the bacterial Eastern Equine Encephalitis germ that infected me. He swears it could not have come from the dead cat in his lab. I suppose if we had any horses on our farm, or if our neighbors had any horses, or if there were any horses within several miles of our farm, then I would agree with him. There weren't any.

Back to present day at the surgery center and the questioning continues. "Have you ever had any reaction to anesthesia? Do you have Diabetes? Are you allergic to any medications?" These are the standard questions they have to ask. They have to know if you might react badly to the anesthesia medications. Diabetics have trouble healing and that needs to be anticipated. I understand the need for these questions.

I wish they would ask some other questions. Like maybe, "Are you scared to die? Did you make out a will so your family will have an easier time dealing with the business end of your death? Do you think you will go to Heaven if you die? How do you feel about your family and friends going on in life after you're gone?" I suppose these are the questions you have to ask, and answer, for yourself.

There are three ways to get rid of cancer: surgery, radiation, and chemotherapy. Holistic health practitioners will tell you about some other methods. I will not tell you they are wrong. Maybe they are right. I got rid of mine with surgery, radiation, and chemotherapy. Each person with cancer has to choose their own treatment path from what is available.

Chapter Five: Surgery

If possible, your doctor will have you undergo surgery to remove the cancerous tissues. Get some rest before the surgery. You may be nervous about the procedure but trust that the surgeon has done a lot of surgeries before and will do well with yours. Remember, surgeons do surgery all the time. He or she knows what they are doing or they would not touch you. Any lawyer will be glad to tell you why.

Surgeons do not mind passing difficult patients off to a more experienced colleague. If you get comfortable with your doctor and then they want to refer you to someone else, trust that the new doc is the one for the job even if you do not like them personally as well as the first doc. You are not trying to make new friends here. You are trying to survive.

After surgery, rest. Remember all those times when you wished you could take a nap in the afternoon and were just too busy? Now you are not too busy. In fact, a nap should be the first thing on your priority list.

And all those friends and family members that call you with some daily drama episode? Tell them you will get back to them next year. Now is the time to take care of yourself, not everyone else.

The morning of my surgery arrives. It's a sunny Tuesday in late October. I have to be at the hospital by 06:30 am. I have a bad habit of being late but not today. There's nothing else on my to-do list this morning, this afternoon, or for that matter, the next week. Surgery in big letters is all the schedule has on it for this date. The pages of the schedule book for next few days are, as they say, left blank on purpose.

I check-in with the receptionist who asks if I know my surgery had been moved to the afternoon. What? No. They tried to call my house last night but I stayed in the valley rather than up at my home in the mountains. You'd think in this day and age that they would see on the computer screen that there is a cell phone number listed along with the home number. They didn't. The protocol says to attempt to contact the patient at home. It doesn't say attempt to contact the patient using any available phone numbers. The worker who wants to get off work on time does just what they are supposed to do and no more. A message was left at the home number. It's my fault I didn't check the machine. Oh well, I couldn't imagine anyone had left me any important messages that couldn't wait until after surgery.

At that moment, a retired minister I've known for the past several years came into the waiting room. I thought I had noticed his car in the parking lot that morning but I didn't think about it really being him. He is the kindest man I've ever met. He cared for a wife with Alzheimer's for many years past the point of her being able to recognize who he was. That is what the phrase, "in sickness and in health" from the traditional marriage vows is all about.

"Came by to see how things were going," he said cheerfully. A quick explanation of the mix up and we are off to share breakfast for him and coffee for me at a nearby restaurant. If you want to be successful in the restaurant business, spend the money to buy a lot near a hospital. The world will beat a path to your door.

We talked. We prayed. We laughed. We cried a little. Cancer makes you appreciate all of these events a little more than you might ever have before. As I said in Chapter one, when you have cancer you find out right away who your friends are. I was sitting with one that morning I didn't know I had.

Same thing happened on my cell phone the night before surgery. I got a message from a guy I used to work with 14 years earlier. He had leukemia about 10 years before my diagnosis and survived. He left the following words of wisdom for me:

"Rick, I heard you are having surgery tomorrow and I wanted to call and wish you the best. When I was going through my cancer treatments, I always went in to the clinic laughing and telling jokes. Everyone would say, "Are you crazy or something? You have leukemia," and I would tell them, "I'm already physically compromised. There isn't anything you are going to do to me today that will hurt me more than the cancer. In fact, what you are going to do to me today is supposed to help me. Why wouldn't I be happy and excited about that?" If you will go into your treatments and clinic visits with that attitude Rick, it will help you. Call me if you need to talk anytime."

I took that advice to heart. When I returned to the surgery clinic, I had a smile on my face, was quick with the jokes, and let them help me. An IV insertion and a pill to make me calm were followed by an injection that was supposed to put me to sleep. I was taken by gurney into the operating room and transferred onto the operating table. I glanced at the clock as I was leaving the prep room: 1:00 pm.

When I was placed on the operating table, the nurse looked at me and said in a stern tone, "He's still awake." I watched as another injection was prepared.

"What are you giving me?" I asked.

"Just some Versed," was the answer. Midazolam, the generic name used "in the business," is a drug that makes you forget. A procedure can be done on you while you are under the influence of midazolam and you will swear that it never happened. I've given it many times in my work and never had problems. That comforted me just then. And with a flick of her wrist on the syringe plunger, I was out.

I open my eyes in the recovery room. It is 4:30

pm. There is a nurse who is male standing beside me. "How you doin'?" he asks.

My throat is extremely sore. More so than it's ever been. I look at him and open my mouth. A muffled "OK" is all I can muster at the moment. I am comforted again to know that I can talk. This means the cancer had not spread to my vocal chords and they did not have to be removed.

Hanging from the ceiling nearby is an LED sign that is connected to a computerized monitoring system. Each patient in the recovery area has a bedside monitor that records the heart rhythm, pulse rate, respiration rate, and blood pressure. The monitors are connected to a central computer that displays any alarm messages on the LED screen. This allows the nurses to see when there is a problem with another patient or if they aren't at the bedside, a problem with their own patient.

An audible alarm dings loudly. I look up and see the LED screen flashing "Apnea alarm bed 7." Apnea, another one of those ten-dollar words, simply means, "not breathing."

I decide to take a deep breath in honor of the moment. It fills my lungs and feels good. My throat is hurting but I can breath. Breathing is the number one most important task your body must perform. You can live for weeks without food, days without water, but you can only live a few precious moments without oxygen.

A few minutes pass and the LED sign again flashes, "Apnea alarm bed 7." I take another deep breath and again, it feels good. I look up at my nurse and glance over at my bedside monitor. "Don't worry about the monitor," he says quickly. He doesn't notice that I'm watching the LED screen.

"What bed is this?" I ask.

"Lucky number seven," he quips.

I fall back asleep. A loud dinging sound awakens me. I look up at the LED screen. It says again, "Apnea alarm bed 7." This happens over and over throughout the afternoon. Each time, I take a few deep breaths and the dinging stops.

It's getting later and the nurse offers me some juice. I know from my own nursing work that he wants to find out if I can swallow. I can but it hurts. I don't say much about the pain. He might not let me go home if I do.

I have a personal theory about pain that allows me a fairly high pain tolerance. My belief is that pain is a signal from the body to the brain that says, "Hey, we've got trouble down here." The brain then responds in ways we don't consciously recognize. Cellular resources are called to emergency status. The engineering department develops a plan to fix the problem. The body's own freeway system, the blood circulatory system, is used to transport materials to the injured area. These materials act as repair technicians, working feverishly to correct, mend, fix, and otherwise alleviate the issue that is causing the pain.

When you take pain meds, the pain stops. The brain then says, "Gosh I'm glad that doesn't hurt anymore. Guess I can call off the reinforcements and use those resources somewhere else." Then when the pain returns, "Why is that still hurting? I thought we fixed that." And the whole system has to go back into repair mode until the signal comes that the pain has stopped. This is why I rarely take any pain medication.

The ride home after surgery is never pleasant for anyone. Whatever got cut on in the operating room is going to feel every bump in the road, every pothole, every quick acceleration, and every sudden stop. Railroad tracks are probably the worst. You endure it. You're glad to be going home. Complain too much and whoever is driving you home might take you back to the hospital.

When I got home, there were two things I knew I had to do: breathe and drink fluids. I had been to the grocery store and bought several flavors of Popsicle® and sorbet. I'm lactose intolerant so the old school treatment, eating ice cream after a tonsillectomy, wasn't going to work for me. As sore as my throat was, hydration was going to be a challenge. I already knew from the LED screen that breathing might be an issue as well.

The best way to judge if you are drinking enough fluids in your life is to think about how much urine you are making. It you are well hydrated, you will need to pee once in a while. The urine will be pale yellow or clear, with either color being fine. If you notice that you have gone hours and hours without needing to urinate and when you do, the urine is a dark amber color, you are already dehydrated.

The day of surgery, the risk for poor hydration is not so bad because during the event, you get intravenous fluids. Sometimes lots of them. This helps keep your blood pressure up. The big risk was going to be the day after. And so it was.

Wednesday morning arrives early enough. I would try to eat as many of the frozen Popsicles and sorbet cups I had stashed in the refrigerator as I could but swallowing was extremely painful. I'm planted on the couch with no intention of moving more than I have to. I eat a bit of the cold stuff but hours go by and I still don't feel like I need to get up to the bathroom. Uh oh.

When you are a nurse, you know too much about what can go wrong with you. A bricklayer might, after surgery, drink a little fluid, not think too much about not having to urinate or how long it has been, and still do just fine. Nurses on the other hand have learned that poor fluid intake can result in kidney failure, stress on all the bodies systems, and if not corrected, certain death. We've seen it all. Dealt with it all. All of it being with someone else.

Now it's me, Nurse Rick, that may have

something go tragically wrong. This is one of those moments when you make a decision that impacts the rest of your life. I decided at that moment that I really wanted to live. To do that, I was going to have to stay hydrated. I decided that eating and drinking was not about the taste anymore. It was about survival. I knew I had to eat and take in liquids in order to survive so I made sure that I did. Whatever it took, I was going to swallow the food and fluids despite the pain, despite the soreness, and despite the fact that the doctor said I would probably end up with a feeding tube coming out of my stomach.

The doctors wanted to put a feeding tube in my stomach before the treatments started. I refused. They said, "But you are a nurse and know what to expect. You know how important nutrition is and you know how to take care of a feeding tube."

My reply was, "The best thing about having cancer is that I am a nurse and I know what to expect. The worst about having cancer is that I am a nurse and I know what to expect."

I asked if anyone ever goes through the treatments without a feeding tube and without losing the ability to swallow. They said that some patients do and I said, "OK, that will be me." I was determined not to lose the ability to swallow. Here is what I did about that problem.

Throat cancer patients often say they cannot swallow food. "It just will not go down," they lament. I learned from another throat cancer survivor that the way to swallow food when your throat does not seem to work is to take a drink of water along with the food. Take a bite of food, take a drink of water. Over time, I could eat without taking water with each bite but for months and months, I drank glass after glass of water with each meal. Whatever it took. I had to do it or I would die.

    First and foremost, you have to keep swallowing despite the fact that it is very painful. Of the many things your body can do, swallowing is right up there at the top of the importance list. I quickly began to rely on a medication that you swish around in your mouth and swallow that is a combination of nystatin and viscous lidocaine. The nystatin kills the thrush bacteria which will develop in your mouth and throat during the treatments and the lidocaine numbs the throat so that it does not hurt to swallow. I used this medication about every four hours for several months. My throat was so sore that it literally would have been too painful to swallow without this concoction.

    I could be wrong about this but I think that the feeding tube would have kept me from swallowing. You see, with the tube, I would not have to swallow. I could just hook up the feeding bag, pour in a substance that looked just like melted milkshake, and the nutrition would just flow into my stomach. No problem. Except for the fact that if I do not have a choice, if I have to swallow to stay alive, I am much more motivated to fight the pain, retrain the muscles in my throat, or do whatever it is that I have to do to keep swallowing.

Would a feeding tube have made it easier? You bet. Would I get one if I had it to do over? Not a chance.

Chapter Six: Radiation

After surgery to remove as much of the cancer as possible, you still have a lot of work to do. Next on the agenda is either radiation or chemotherapy or both. HMOs have something called a Tumor Board, a group of medical personnel, who look over your case and decide what treatment you need. You never meet them. You do not know who they are. You do not even know what type of medical people are on the board. But they know your case. And your fate. How do they know your fate? They decide it.

For me, both radiation of the neck and a course of chemotherapy were advised. This is probably because I was otherwise healthy and could stand both treatments. These are not easy things to endure.

Radiation involves laying on a table in a room with a big machine that looks like some kind of scanner device in a science fiction movie. Actually, it is. It sends out radio waves at your body that are focused on the area of your cancer. It moves around and sends the beams at you from different directions. This takes about ten minutes for most cancers. Head and neck areas are more difficult and they require two sessions back to back thus making the treatment just over twenty minutes.

Radiation is not too bad if you do not need it done on your head or neck, which of course is exactly where I had to have it. The new multi-beam radiation machines can be programmed to hit tumors with better accuracy than before and they are affordable enough that smaller hospitals have them.

For head and neck cancers, the big problem is keeping your head and neck in the right position for the radiation beams to hit you. In order to do that, my head had to be held on to the radiation table by a custom made mask. Think Jason from the "Friday the 13th" series of horror films.

If you happen to be claustrophobic, you are in serious trouble. I thought that since I often wore a motorcycle helmet this part of the equation would be a piece of cake. Not so. The first time I was secured to the table with the mask, I quickly realized just how long the twenty-two minute treatment was going to take.

It was awful. I felt trapped and in fact, I was. You cannot get up, you cannot roll over, and in that position with a sore throat, you cannot swallow. Of course the radiation is going to burn out your saliva glands, so really you are not going to have to swallow anyway but then there is the side effect of dry mouth that not having any saliva glands brings and you cannot get up to get a drink no matter how dry your throat gets. I knew I had to endure the time but thankfully it was made much easier by a helpful radiation tech.

Each day, the radiation tech would be

responsible for strapping me down to the table and making sure the body alignment was correct before disappearing to the control room to start the machine. On the first day of treatment, the tech tried to reassure me by saying that he would be watching me from the control room via a camera and that if I felt I need to, I could raise my hand and he would stop the treatment and come unstrap me from the table.

While that is reasonable and offered me some comfort about the possibility of a panic attack, I knew truthfully that if I became sick and regurgitated while in that position I would likely drown before he could get back in the room and unstrap me and sit me up. Sometimes you just have to tell yourself that something is not going to happen. I try to follow such self-proclamations with a prayer for help from above. I never did throw-up and die on the radiation table. I am thankful to God to this day that I did not.

As the tech was leaving the room, he asked calmly if I would like a little music to help me get through the treatment.

I immediately said "Yes" being so into music as I am. I was already secured to the table so I could not see him sift through a stack of CDs, select one, put it the boom box across the room, and press play.

All of a sudden, the boom box started blaring screaming loud alternative rock at about 110 decibels. I had been expecting maybe a little smooth jazz or something new age since this was California but no, I was being bombarded with loud music that I did not recognize.

Then something caught my ear. "Was that a late beat on the drums? Did the drummer do that intentionally? What the heck is he going to do next?"

I listened intensely to the next song to see if the drummer did that same thing again. "The late beat had been a mistake, no doubt. "I darn sure would not have played it that way," I thought to myself. The song after that came and went and then another and another. Suddenly the tech came back into the room, turned off the boom box, and unstrapped my facemask.

"Are we done already?" I asked.

"That's twenty-two minutes. You're done." he replied.

That is when I realized that the obscure music, a band I would have never picked myself, loud and obnoxious, was in fact the perfect distraction. "The music was just right. I did not even realize the time was going by so quickly," I told him.

The tech looked at me and said simply, "Tomorrow, bring your own CD if you like. Anything you want, loud as you want. Whatever it takes to get you through these treatments."

I already knew from listening to music during

dental procedures that the worst thing to do is bring your favorite CD. You do not want to do that because then you associate that music with a painful procedure and that is not what you want for your favorite music.

I went through my CD collection that night and picked out music that would be fast paced, with loud electric guitar and good drum grooves, but something I would not mind never listening to again. I already knew that after the radiation treatments were over, I would put the CD away and never, ever, listen to it again.

And that is just what I did. There were a few days that I took something else for a little variety but mostly I kept that same CD. It had over an hour of music so I technically was not listening to the same songs day after day even though the CD was the same. That did it for me most days. Then there was Lou.

In my opinion, the finest voice in the history of rock music is the original lead singer with the group Foreigner. His name is Lou Gramm and after leaving Foreigner, he had a successful solo career. A few years ago, he was diagnosed with a brain tumor and went through a rough treatment and recovery period. I attended several of his concerts when he returned to the stage and it was obvious he did not feel well.

But there he was, singing for all he was worth, fronting a band, earning money doing what he had always done. That says something. That says strength, determination, and perseverance. I would listen to Lou's CDs on some treatment days when I was feeling low and I needed some of that strength, determination, and perseverance for myself.

Lou played at a local casino one night during my treatments. I went to hear him even though I really did not feel very good. He sounded the best that night that I had ever heard. He had done it. He had recovered, had his voice back in good shape, and as we say, rocked the house. I left that night knowing that if he could do it, then so could I. When you have cancer, find your hope wherever it suits you best. Just find it.

Music helped my spirit get through radiation. You will need a few other things to get your skin through it.

Your skin will look sunburned where the radiation hits you but you will be alive. For the sunburn-like irritation, I found that pure aloe vera lotion helped. You can find it at the health food store and look for a "pure" brand with no perfumes. The perfumes just irritate your skin even more.

I put this on the area of my skin that was being radiated every day after my treatment. I did not leave the radiation treatment room until I had put on my aloe vera. I know the cancer treatment unit is busy but hey, this is my skin, my time for treatment, and I made sure I took the extra two minutes to take care of myself and put that aloe vera on my face before getting out in the sun and wind. If I do not make sure I am taken care of properly, who will?

During the weeks of treatment with radiation, I came to a time when the aloe vera did not help anymore. I could tell the very day that it happened that my skin was too dry. It may have been my own fault.

While going through treatments, I would try to have one errand to run while I was coming home from the clinic. One errand was really all I had the energy for but I would make sure I had that one thing to do so I would push myself to do as much as I could and not lose even more strength and determination.

One day, that errand was to go to the cell phone store and have something or other done to my phone. I really do not remember what was needed but my treatments were early in the morning at that time and I had arrived at the store about 20 minutes prior to opening time. I sat in my truck, listening to music, and did not realize that the left side of my face was in the bright sunlight. Several minutes went by and all of a sudden that side of my face felt very hot and dry. I knew I had messed up but other than scoot over out of the sunlight, I could not do anything else about it right then. You have to stay aware during cancer treatments. You can mess up and do something that hurts you very quickly and not even realize that it is happening.

If you do mess something up though, you still

have to keep going. There is no choice really. The next day after my treatment, I saw the doctor and was prescribed Biafine cream, a prescription-only med that carried me through the remainder of my treatments quite well with no further skin damage.

Here is something else you can do if your radiation involves the head and neck. Go buy an orange shirt or blouse. When you wear that color up around your face, you do not look as red and sunburned. This will make you feel better about yourself when you are out in public.

When you have head and neck radiation, I think the most important thing is retaining the ability to swallow. Besides minimizing the pain of swallowing with the nystatin/lidocaine mixture, another part of continuing to swallow is keeping your throat stretched out. I took some singing lessons once and learned a few warm-up exercises as part of my vocal studies. One of those exercises involved opening up the throat by singing a note that starts on a medium pitch and then sliding down to a very low pitch. That stretches your throat and helps prevent scar tissue from building up and preventing you from swallowing. I did that exercise at least twice a day during treatments and still continue to do it to this day. Scar tissue can build-up for years after the treatments end and keeping the throat stretched out is key to continuing to be able to swallow. I would faithfully do the exercise while walking back to my pick-up truck after the treatments.

Once inside the truck, there was one more thing I would do to help promote swallowing. I would drive a few blocks to a local Der Weinersnitzel fast food drive-in and buy the cheap combo meal with two hot dogs. Hot dogs are not exactly health food mind you, but there is a reason for this choice. Radiation and chemotherapy change your taste buds and food does not taste the same as it used to. Often times, everything has a metallic taste that is not very pleasant. For a while, things got really wacky and I would be eating one thing and it would taste like something else. I distinctly remember drinking a soda one day and thinking that it tasted like melted ice cream. Very strange.

That of course was right before I lost all ability to drink soda. It simply burned too much. Spicy foods had to go as well; too painful. French fries? No more. Too hard to swallow somehow. And the biggest loss for me? Ketchup. I suppose it was the vinegar in it that made it burn but it did indeed burn and did so for many, many months. Even several years after treatment, I can only eat small amounts of ketchup without it burning my taste buds.

But throughout my treatments, for some odd reason hot dogs retained their taste and were somehow more delicious than ever. I made a deal with myself that, if I could get through the radiation treatment without raising my hand to stop, I would treat myself with a hot dog afterward. I never had to raise my hand. It was not always a hot dog that I would eat, but mostly it was. I believe this routine kept my throat in motion and thereby helped me keep swallowing. To this day, when I eat certain foods, I remember how good they tasted when almost nothing else did. Hot dogs, salmon, and honey-baked ham kept me alive for a long time.

When you are going through cancer treatments, my advice is to immediately stop smoking and drinking alcohol. Period. Your liver is going to be busy enough with the all work it has to do to process the toxins in your treatments. Beside, you knew you needed to do this anyway, right? Now you have to. It might be tough at first but remember, the cancer is going to change your life for the better. This might just be one way it does that.

You will feel more tired as the radiation treatments continue. Frequent naps are OK. If you need someone to drive you to treatments, do not be shy about asking. I drove myself right up to the end but it was my daily project to do so and was all I did during the final few treatments.

The best advice my surgeon gave me was, "Listen to your body." If you are tired, nap. If you are hungry, eat. If you are not making much urine, drink even if you are not thirsty. You body is telling you it is thirsty in a different way. Bored? Find something to do. Listen to your body. It will not lie to you about what it needs.

Chapter Seven: Chemotherapy

Chemotherapy presents a different set of challenges from the radiation. Chemotherapy is a fancy word for chemical therapy. Called chemo for short, it involves poisoning you. Yes, you are about to be poisoned. The idea behind this treatment is to make every cell in your body sick. The weak cancerous ones will die and the others will survive and return to health.

Once an intravenous line inserted and the nurse gets your chemo fluids hung, you have at least a four-hour process to endure while the various fluids are infusing into your veins. I received saline for hydration, some albumin, and a large dose of chemo during each of my three chemotherapy sessions. These things take time to infuse.

The chemo nurse's advice? Bring a lunch. You are going to be here for a while.

The chemotherapy treatment area can be a sad place. The other patients are either like me, just starting the process, or like the patient next to me, curled up on the recliner in fetal position, sleeping, enduring what may be the last days of his life. "Not going there," I kept reminding myself.

I believe that you are what you read. I would take magazines along with my food and fluids. I was determined to get back to riding and would spend my chemo time reading travel stories, reviews of new motorcycles, and anything that would give me a sense that there was going to be life left to live and the strength left to live it.

How many times have you heard the old saying, "Stay away from that guy. He is just a dreamer." I am here to tell you that I do not automatically think that is a bad thing. Sometimes in your life, and several times in my life, dreams are all you have to go on. Turning dreams into reality may take some doing but remember that the reality you seek started with someone's dream. When you are sitting in a recliner in a chemotherapy treatment suite with an intravenous line pouring poison into your veins, dreams are all you have.

Cells that change a lot, like hair cells, are impacted the most. That is why many people lose their hair during chemo treatments. I kept most of my hair by cutting my pony tail short to remove the weight and then on the day of chemo and for a couple of days after, I did not wash my hair or pull on it very hard. Sure it did not look so great but there is no beauty contest going on down at the cancer treatment center. Go in there with greasy hair that is barely combed. It is just hair.

The other problem with chemotherapy is nausea. This gets almost everyone that goes through chemo. I found a trick that worked and I share it every chance I get.

On the day of chemo, they will give you anti-nausea medications. Lots of them. Then they will tell you to take a usual dose of the meds every eight hours for three to five days after the treatment. For my first chemo treatment, this really did not help very much.

Just before the second treatment, I was feeling nauseated one day and almost threw up in the kitchen sink in front of my nephew who was visiting me. I remember seeing the look in his eye; a look of fear that he did not know how to help me. I saw the anti-nausea meds on the kitchen counter and thought to myself, "I am a nurse. I know these meds will help me. Just take them and do not scare anyone anymore."

I asked the chemo doctor if it was alright to do this and he said, "You are a nurse. I know you will not take too much. Go ahead." For the three days prior to my second treatment, I took the anti-nausea meds every eight hours and did feel better. What really mattered though is when the second dose of chemo was complete, I did not get as nauseated. I did just a little bit but I was not throwing up all over like the first time.

I did the same regimen for my third chemo dose and sure enough, it worked again. I told the chemo doc about this and he said, "Your chemo drug, Cysplatin, makes everyone sick. You may have found a new protocol for us to use." I hope that is true. I hope I never have to use it again though.

Also remember that nausea is a hydration problem. If you feel nauseated, drink fluids. Sounds like the opposite advice you would usually hear but it works. If you notice that you are not urinating as often as you usually would, you are getting dehydrated. Drink. If this is not enough, go to the chemo nurses and ask them to give you a liter of normal saline through an IV. How much better you will feel is worth the needle stick.

Radiation and chemotherapy can lower your appetite. Your need for good nutrition is very high during this time. Proteins are necessary to help repair and regenerate the normal cells in the area being treated while calories are needed to give you extra energy. If you find that you do not want to eat, have the doctor prescribe a medication called Megace. This med is actually pregnant female hormones. Yes, it is true. The med will increase your appetite sufficiently but you may find yourself crying over a romantic movie or an old song you hear on the radio. Do not ask me how I know.

Another important tip is to avoid crowds and large stores while you are in treatment for cancer. Your immune system will be on break for a while. Do not put yourself at risk for viruses and bacteria that are going around.

Wearing a surgical mask over your nose and mouth might help but I do not like to do that. When you have one of those masks on, you are really only avoiding large droplet-based particles, like from someone sneezing nearby. Unless it is form-fitted to your face, like a military gas mask, you are still breathing in unfiltered air around its edges. I think it makes you breath in a lot of carbon dioxide from your own exhaled breath as well. Combine these problems with the fact that many viruses and bacteria are picked up from surfaces by contact with your hands and you can understand why I do not think the surgical mask is a magic answer. Avoid crowds and large stores. It is not that hard to do for a few months.

Chapter Eight: Dark Days

If you have cancer, there will be some dark days. I am going to share with you two of my darkest days but I am just doing so in an attempt to show you that you can get through them. It is not fun when dark days happen. But you will get through them if you try.

The first was three days after my surgery. I am home alone. I can barely swallow at all. I finally get a flashlight and look at my throat because it feels like something is wrong in there. Sure enough, I have a large piece of skin or something hanging down in my throat that is irritating me every time I try to swallow.

I called the clinic that did my surgery and the nurse said that this happens sometimes and it will just fall off by itself. When? They cannot say, of course. I decided I would try to cut it out myself. That plan lasted only a short time. I sterilized, best I could, a pair of tweezers and scissors. I could not hold the light, the tweezers, and the scissors all at one time. I dropped the whole setup in the sink accidentally, thus contaminating everything beyond what I knew I could clean up. It is off to the Emergency Room for me at 10pm on a Friday night, the worst possible time to visit any ER, anywhere.

The Kaiser ER is no exception that night. The

young doctor on duty goes by protocol and has one of the Ear, Nose, and Throat clinic docs look me over. "It will fall off by itself. Do not clip it," is the advice his supervisor gives him. He is a young resident and does not want to do anything without approval of the department chief. He runs off to go to another patient and the ER doctor takes mercy on me and clips it anyway.

Relieved, I go back home to sleep. It still hurts to swallow but at least I am not gagging every time I try to do so.

The other dark day involves the other end of my body. When you have chemotherapy, one of two things is going to happen to your colon. You are either going to get diarrhea or constipation. My colon went the way of constipation.

It is a manageable problem if you try to manage it. So far, I had not. At first, I did not realize it was happening so I did not know to do anything. A little more medical knowledge for you: your colon's real job is to absorb water. Huh? Yeah, that is right. A lot of water is reabsorbed into the body from the slurry your small intestine dumps into your large intestine, otherwise known as the colon. That is why when something goes wrong in the colon, you might have the watery output commonly known as diarrhea. Stuff moved through the colon too fast and none of the water was removed. Or you might have constipation. Stuff moved through the colon too slowly and too much water was removed. Now it is like concrete and nothing is going anywhere.

How do you fix constipation quickly? Put some more water up in there. That is what an enema does.

One night, my constipation is so bad that I am physically hurting inside. As a nurse, I know I need an enema, which I can buy at the local pharmacy. Problem is the local pharmacy, when you live in a small mountain community, is a half-hour drive away.

I make my way out to my pick-up truck and drive down the hill. It is the middle of the night but I do not care because I am in a painful situation and I know something has to be done. I visit two locations before I find an open pharmacy. Then it is back up the hill to my home to self-administer the enema.

Now another hour of pain has gone by and I am desperate. I am lying on the bathroom floor trying to give myself the enema and get some relief. It is your lowest day in life when you are lying on the bathroom floor, crying, hurting, trying to give yourself an enema.

When relief finally comes, there is blood in my stool. That can happen with chemotherapy too. I continued to have small amounts of blood in my stool until the chemotherapy was completed. I watched carefully to make sure I was not losing too much blood and I never did.

Now here is the good part. That is as low as it

gets. Whatever your lowest days entail, you can find a way through them. For me, I had to visit the emergency room on a Friday night and I had to drive an hour to the store and back then give myself an enema. How bad is that? Bad enough. But manageable.

If you feel like the dark days are taking over, go to your doctor and ask for an antidepressant medication. At the advice of my favorite Kaiser physician, I took Prozac for several months. When this drug first came on the market, it gained some negative publicity due to several cases of suicide. The problem was that it worked so well, people that were severely depressed and barely functioning in life, began to feel well enough to do themselves in. You are likely not that depressed but how could you have cancer and not be depressed about it? It is OK to be upset about this problem! Take some Prozac and decide to live.

Chapter Nine: Christmas and Cancer

I was raised in a rural Christian home where weekly church services were rarely missed and nightly prayers for family and friends went up faithfully. We were taught to respect all races and creeds. We were schooled in family history and the history of our state and country. We learned to respect nature, to harvest the fruit of the land, and to love.

We also learned about war. I used to watch the nightly news to hear the kill rates for Vietcong vs. American soldiers during the Vietnam War era. How sad to think that the numbers were always skewed by the authorities to make it look like our side was winning. I hung on every word the newsman would say about the war. Of course it was never really a declared war, just "The Vietnam Conflict" but we knew. People don't die when two governments are conflicted. People die when those governments go to war with each other. Whether the paperwork is done to make the problem a declared war or not, the soldiers, and more than a few innocent bystanders, are just as dead.

Back in the day, as we say, Christmas represented a time of hope. As a child, you could hope for a certain gift that you had seen on television or in a magazine. You had to be good all year or Santa Claus might not come by with it. What a ploy by the parents that concept is. Good all year? No one can meet that goal. Your sibling or a neighbor kid or a relative, somebody, is going to irritate the living fire right out of you one day and you are going to say or do something about it that rubs someone the wrong way, irritates them or your parents or whoever is in charge of you at that moment, and gets you in trouble.

Temporary punishments are tolerable. The physical pain of getting your butt whipped, the humiliation of standing alone in a corner, or the solitude of a timeout period will quickly end. You can stand those things. But the thought that you might have just blown Christmas, that Santa Claus was in the North Pole right now marking your name on the naughty list, was devastating. As the old song says, "You better not pout, you better not cry, you better be good… Santa Claus is coming to town," and he might not come visit you while he is here if you do not straighten up.

Because we went to church, I knew the truth about Christmas early on. There is no Santa Claus (sorry to burst your bubble) but there is a Jesus. You should be good because this guy gave his life to prove the point that there is continued life after death. I wonder at the miracles he performed and embrace his teachings that promote meekness. The meek may inherit the earth, according to the Bible, but it seems to me that the evil, mean people have a pretty good hold on it at the moment.

Though I believe meekness is a true virtue, everyone experiences the four core emotions at some point: happy, sad, anger, and fear. There's no escaping these four. Every other emotion, like jealousy and envy for example, is some combination of those four.

Jealousy of your lover's best friend means you are sad that this person spends time with your lover that could be your time and that you are scared this friend might mean something to your lover that you cannot compete with. Sadness combined with fear equals jealousy.

Envy is related to jealousy in that you are sad that your neighbor has a new BMW and you don't, and you are scared that you might not ever have a new BMW or that your car could breakdown soon leaving you stranded. Something that new BMW just couldn't ever do, no sir, no way. My neighbor will never be standing in the hot summer sun, dying of thirst, no breeze blowing, out of breath, kicking the side of a broken down car. No sir. I hate that neighbor, don't you? Sadness, fear, and anger equals envy.

Even Jesus lost it one time and wrecked the money exchange market. Seems the locals in charge of exchanging currency types were overcharging the public. I wonder what Jesus would think of ATM out of network usage fees?

How easily our emotions are aroused. Christmas and Easter arouse special emotions.

Peace. Goodwill. Kindness. Thoughtfulness. Reverence. Hope for a nice life after death, proven for the first time by the fact that Jesus showed up in front of some of his biggest fans after he died. If some Elvis fans had said they saw Elvis after he died, we would question their sanity. But Jesus was different. Somebody says they saw him after he died and the story gets told for 21 centuries. And all of this without a tour bus, stage lighting, or a 10,000-watt sound system. No satellite up-link, no DirectTV® Pay Per View Special, not even a Yahoo home page hyperlink. Makes you wonder how the guy got any notoriety at all doesn't it? I'll have to get the cell phone out and call his personal assistant to get the name of his marketing people. They're awesome aren't they?

Other holidays bring up different emotions. In the United States, the Fourth of July brings out patriotism, love of country, triumph of spirit. Memorial Day and Presidents Day carry these same emotions in progressively lesser degrees. Halloween? Fear. Thanksgiving is a mix of church and state. We are thankful to God for our blessings but the holiday was established by the government to honor the survival of the Pilgrims.

Of all the holidays, my favorite is definitely Christmas. Why? I think it is the sense of peace that comes over the planet on that day. Decades ago that peace stretched over more days but now that Wal-Mart only closes for that lone 24 hour period, the feeling is shorter. It's like the world stops to take a deep breath, maybe sigh a little, and start refreshed, ready to return unwanted gifts the next morning. We need that peace. It is the opposite of war and we certainly have plenty of that.

I had cancer during Christmas. Two things stood out to me as I prepared to face that reality. One was that I would probably be around family and they would have to see me sick. I did not mind so much because I could not do anything about it. I had cancer. I cannot change that for the Christmas family get-together. But I would have to see them, their faces, and feel their attitudes about me. More emotion I did not need.

Second was my concern about food. Holiday meals are a special event meant to be enjoyed. I was particularly happy that I would be getting ham since I had discovered that the chemo did not kill the taste of that particular treat. In fact, the flavor was enhanced somehow and ham tasted like candy. I would enjoy that but I knew I could not eat very much. My appetite was poor and everyone would be pushing me to eat more because they would not understand. Besides the poor appetite, when it hurts to swallow, you only want to eat as much food as you need to survive.

Then there is that funny feeling you get when you contemplate whether this might be your last Christmas. This was not so much of a concern for me because I had made up my mind to live. But then again, was it my choice to live or God's kind indulgence that would allow me to survive this? I believe it is a combination of both and I knew I would see other Christmas seasons. I would never have guessed how great some of them to come might be.

Chapter Ten: Recovery Phase: I Am Alive!

The doctors and techs said that during the last week of radiation treatments and chemo, I would probably be too weak to drive myself to the treatment center. On the last day of radiation, when I left the building and got into my pickup truck to drive myself back home, I kept thinking to myself, "I did it. It's over."

Now what? Now it is time to heal, gain strength, and start getting back to life. But how? The effects of the radiation treatments carry on for several weeks after the actual treatment sessions stop. So does the tiredness.

My routine for several weeks was to wake up, eat a small breakfast, clean up the breakfast dishes, clean myself up with a shower, then go back to bed for a mid-morning nap. I would wake up about noon and make some lunch, which I would eat while watching funny cartoons favorites from my childhood. After cleaning up the lunch dishes, then it was back to bed for my afternoon nap. I would get up for dinner and stay awake during the evening but had no trouble falling back to sleep at a reasonable bedtime. The next day the process was repeated.

This sounds like a lot of sleep if you have never had chemo and radiation. If you have, you know I am on to something good here.

Sleep is when the body heals. The energy it takes to be awake, up walking around, thinking, doing things, eating and drinking, is a lot. When you sleep, none of that is going on so the chemical processes necessary for healing can take priority over everything else. If you do not think this is true, then why are you tired when you go to sleep and refreshed when you wake up? And if you do not wake up refreshed, it is because you do not sleep well, right? Well then it is settled. The body heals while it sleeps.

I balance all that sleep with another thing that I think is essential to healing. On the weekends, I suggest that even if you are tired, get out and go somewhere and do something. Go to a movie, or a live play, or a sporting event, or a concert. It is even better if you have to go out of town for this and stay overnight.

Why do all this on weekends when sleeping was the advice for the weekdays? You need stimulation and good feelings. Start with a movie. That is the easiest. There is no work to be done at all to see a movie except for just sitting there and sipping your water. All those snacks you were trying to stay away from before, well you need the calories now. Enjoy them. Where do you think your body gets the energy to heal itself? And you probably just lost a lot of weight during the treatments. Stimulate your brain with a good movie and stimulate your taste buds with something sweet to eat. Not a bad way to spend a couple of hours.

Move up over time to a weekend get away. You do not have to do anything elaborate. Just go somewhere new. Eat at a restaurant you have never been to before. Go to a movie in a different theater. Walk down new streets. Stimulate your brain and your taste buds. I made several trips during my recovery phase and it helped immensely.

Another important part of this whole process of beating cancer involves getting your brain to feel like it is in a better state of mind. Every weekday while I was in treatments and in recovery, I would watch an old cartoon show on DVD that I remembered liking as a child. I had purchased it at the bookstore before I had cancer just because I liked it and it was on sale. Now it was a lifesaver.

The Rocky and Bullwinkle Show, Complete Second Season, was not filled with perfect writing, world-class animation, or anything fancy. It was however, something I had watched as a child and when I would watch it as an adult, I would go back to that place in my mind when I was in a new body, with abundant energy, and good health. I would laugh at the jokes and let myself be happy. Forget the cancer. Remember the childhood health and energy.

If you are a person that did not have health as a child, go back to a time when you were healthy as a younger adult and pick something from that era to watch. All you are trying to do is get some good feelings going in your brain to replace the bad feelings that worry over the cancer, its treatments, and its side effects, will give you. Only you can control how you feel. It is up to you to change how you feel.

Another important thing is to find a project to do. Something that will take time but not necessarily a lot of money or energy. My project was to convert old family photographs into digital picture files.

Growing up, my dad had a 35mm film camera and lots of slide photographs were taken. The family would often set up the projector and load in the slide trays and watch as pictures of past holidays and birthdays went by. It was sort of like a primitive Power Point presentation for those reading this that are too young to remember slide projectors and screens.

I called my dad and asked him to send me all the old family slides so I could save them to the computer using an attachment I had purchased for the digital camera. It held two slides at once and allowed you to shoot a digital picture of the slide, one at a time, then reload. A few days after my request, I received a box with 1200 slides in it. My sister soon sent another box with a few hundred more. The project was a go.

On days when I did not have much energy, I still could sit awhile and shoot a few slides. It did not take much physical energy but it took more mental energy than you might imagine. Managing the large number of slides and corresponding large number of files was not a simple task. Beyond that, there was the mental energy required to simply relive each of these slides as they went by. But again, I must say that this process can take you back to a healthier time. There can be some bad times in reviewing old pictures too but now is the time in your life when you are letting go of all that drama. You are trying to live through cancer and that trumps anything you have ever been through and makes it seem so manageable in comparison.

Watch for cues from Heaven in this process as well. You never know when they are going to come but I am here to tell you, they are coming.

I was shooting slides one day and came across several Sunday School pictures taken on an Easter Sunday morning when I was about 7 years old. Two kids from the next farm over were there in the front row. Slides from the next Easter with some of the same Sunday School kids, including the brother and sister in the first photo, followed. Then one from a birthday party a few years later surfaced with the same brother and sister. I felt compelled to send a copy of these to the mother of my two childhood friends and I did. Almost three years would go by before the significance of this simple act would become evident. Another example of how patience is a virtue.

Now, one more thing. When you lay down for your naps, look up at the ceiling and starting thinking about possibilities. How do you want to spend the rest of your life? If you are beating cancer, and going to live, you do not have to go back to what was before. Want a new job? What job do you really want? Think of how you could get that job. What would it take? Could you feel strong enough tomorrow to make one phone call to start the process rolling? Sure you could.

Want to change where you live? You could do that. Grab some real estate magazines after the next trip over to the radiation suite. Look through the homes for sale or apartments for rent and picture yourself living there. Go through some of your possessions and start packing for the move.

Need to change the people in your life? Now is the time. Those you need to keep are evident. Those you need to let go of are evident too. Pray about it. Consider it carefully. But do not let the chance to change your life pass you by.

Actually, there is not anything you cannot do. You just have to stop telling yourself you cannot do it. One of my favorite remarks that I make whenever someone is expressing a negative opinion about something I want to do is this: "I can think of a hundred ways that this won't work. All I need is one way that it will work and I'll just go with that." Tell yourself that you can change and you will. Tell yourself you cannot, and for sure, you will not.

Recovery is all about change. Not only can you do it, you have to. There really is no other choice.

You may think you do not have enough strength to make changes right now. Do not be concerned. It is coming. You will know when it gets here. I knew the day I picked up a piece of paper and made a list of things I wanted to do on my next trip down the hill into town. I looked at that list and said to myself, "Oh my! I feel like doing more than one thing today."

I have been an avid list maker most of my life. It helps me stay organized. I had not made a list since before my surgery but I caught myself making one that day. I knew then that I was gaining strength. I knew I was feeling better. I knew, deep down inside, that I was going to get over the cancer and start to live again.

Chapter Eleven: The Road to Recovery

Each cancer patient has their own road to follow. My road, literally, was a paved highway.

My sister, whom I love dearly, was turning 50 years old. That is a milestone kind of birthday that deserves celebrating. Her kids, my nieces, decided to have a party for her and I knew I had to go to Iowa where she lives and join in the festivities.

Most cancer recovery-phase patients would have cautiously bought an airline ticket and done everything they could to minimize the effort involved in making the trip from California to the Mid-West.

Not me. I had this theory that pushing myself only made me stronger. That, or maybe I thought that I just was not ready to give up certain things I liked doing, like taking motorcycle trips. The sidecar rig I had purchased just before diagnosis was calling out to me to take a long ride. And so I did.

Now mind you, I was not in the best shape for this trip. I still had radiation damage on my tongue that hurt constantly. My mouth was dry from the radiation and I could barely swallow. I was thin and tired easily. None of this mattered to me. I was going to ride my motorcycle sidecar rig to Iowa and no one could talk me out of it.

That does not mean I was reckless about planning. The first thing I needed to do was gain some strength. Like many people, I had a gym membership I hardly ever used. That needed to change. I started with a few minutes on the typical machines that strengthen your extremities and would end with a few minutes on the treadmill.

The first day, I began to sweat while on the treadmill. Suddenly, I began to smell something that took me a moment to identify. I knew I recognized it but it was out of place. I was smelling the scent of the chemotherapy treatment center. The chemotherapy chemicals were literally coming out of my pores.

All I could think was, "Get this stuff out of me." Each time I worked out, I was happy to sweat the stuff out. How do I know for sure this was the chemo coming out? All I can tell you is that if I showered before I left the gym, I felt fine. If I left without a shower, it felt like the chemicals would reabsorb through my skin and I felt sick the rest of the day. Once I figured out what was happening, I never left the gym without a shower again.

I had a small ice chest that would fit neatly in the sidecar. I packed it with snacks I could tolerate eating and with Ensure for more serious nutrition. I had a CamelBack® water-filled backpack with a hose that allowed me to ride and drink water at the same time. This would help me avoid dehydration and keep my mouth moist. My tongue would hurt more severely if I let my mouth get too dry. I packed clothes for any weather condition that might arise on a cross-country trip in May, which is just about any weather condition possible because in May, anything can happen. And I packed a gift for my sister; some pictures of her from the family slide project.

The day I left was not necessarily a triumphant, throw caution to the wind, kind of day. I had made many motorcycle trips before and knew exactly what to do. This was my first long sidecar trip. That type of bike, while more stable when sitting still, is more difficult to drive than a regular two-wheeled motorcycle. All I knew was that I had to make this trip. I had to prove to myself that I had it in me to persevere.

And I did. I made sure I ate well in the morning and at night. Lunch was lite on the road. I slept well each night so I would have the strength to get up and go again the next day. It snowed on me in Wyoming. Funny thing was I saw another sidecar rig on the road that day, going in the opposite direction I was headed. It gave me hope that I was not crazy for riding in that type of weather.

My sister's birthday was the best. She was surprised to see me but glad too because we are close and I know she worried about the cancer possibly taking me away. It did not though. We are still close to this day.

I stayed a few days with one of my nieces, then visited family and friends down South before heading back to California. I stopped by a motorcycle diner in Dallas made famous in a short-lived TV show called Texas Hardtails. A hardtail is a type of motorcycle that has no rear shock. I had a fried baloney sandwich, a favorite of the shop owner, and thought about getting a tattoo of the ribbon for throat cancer (like the pink ribbon you see for breast cancer, only the colors are different: maroon with a cream-colored border) but decided against it. My health was still not fully recovered and I thought it might be better not to irritate my skin so much.

Did the trip go perfectly? They never do. I had to buy a new rear tire in Odessa. Sidecar rigs are notoriously hard on rear tires. I thought I could make it home on the tire I had but another motorcyclist at a gas station pointed out to me how thin the tread had gotten and I knew I had to do something immediately. I backtracked a few miles to the Harley shop and was soon back on the road with a brand new rear tire.

Riding toward the sunset across the vastness of west Texas, I noticed my tongue had stopped hurting. The trip had done its intended job. I was getting stronger, healthier, and happier.

Chapter Twelve: Chemo Brain

The brain is an organ just like any other. It is a very important, and sensitive, part of your body. All the organs work together to make the body function the way it does but the brain in particular influences life in ways that are both incomparable and paramount.

When the chemotherapy drugs are coursing through your veins, they are coursing through your brain too. There can be an effect on your thinking processes that researchers are just starting to take notice of and substantiate. It is commonly called "Chemo Brain."

Chemo Brain is a loosely defined term that covers any number of alterations in thought and behavior that a chemo patient might display. You might forget things more easily or have trouble remembering details, common words, or dates. Concentration can be difficult. Multitasking near impossible. It seems like everything takes longer than it should. The symptoms can improve over time though some of them may last for years.

How do you treat Chemo Brain? There are not any clear guidelines as yet. My answer was to strive to be methodical, in other words, have a method of doing things and stick with that method every day. In my home, there is a place where all the keys are kept. It is a small bowl in the kitchen and the rule is that when you come in and unload your pockets for the night, all keys go in that spot. Car keys, house keys, office keys, whatever keys, go in that spot. Does this eliminate searching for lost keys? Sadly, no. But it greatly minimizes the occurrence rate of that problem.

This is not a new concept for me. As a professional drummer, I have hauled drums around since I was 12 years old. Drum sets have lots of parts to them; drums, stands, cymbals, sticks, and of course your music. You cannot leave any of this equipment at home or at the venue where you are playing. You cannot leave it because number one, you need it to play, and number two, if you leave it you cannot just go buy another one. Musical instruments tend to be expensive, unique, and very personal so thinking that, "Oh well, I'll just go get a replacement," is not going to work. You have to be careful, meticulous, and thorough when packing up your drums.

Chemo Brain makes you carry that same methodology over into your life. When I am packing my briefcase for work, there are certain things that go in certain places. I can see them there and know I have my things and that I am OK. When I bring mail into the house from the post office, there is a consistent place to put it. If I am looking for something later that I know I saw in the mail, I can find it there. If I do not follow these methods, things just get lost and a frustrating effort has to be made to locate them.

The frustration part of it comes from the concept that you, as a cancer patient, now have a stark understanding of how precious, and finite, time really is. If you are going through treatments or have survived cancer, either way, your concept of the importance of each hour of life is amplified. You want to spend each minute living life, enjoying it, and relishing the time you have. Spending even a few minutes looking for lost keys seems painfully wrong.

How did Chemo Brain affect me most? After my treatments were over, I just did not feel as sharp mentally and my reflexes were off. I went out to my motorcycles one day and made one of those decisions that would change the rest of my life. I thought to myself, "I've had a good run with these bikes. I've ridden many trouble-free miles, traveled all over the country and never had a serious accident. Am I going to keep riding until I do have an accident or am I going to stop now and call it done?" I called it done, sold every bike I owned, even the sidecar rig I rode to my sisters birthday party, and walked away from riding.

Do I miss it? No. Something told me it was time for a change and that God had other plans on the horizon. My music life would soon be returning to me. I just did not know it yet.

Chapter Thirteen: I Don't Do Broken

Here is another thing to watch out for. If you are recovering from cancer, you might find yourself spending a lot of money and I do not mean on medical bills. What may happen to you is that you will come to know the phrase, "I don't do broken."

"I don't do broken" was a catch phrase that became a credo. It meant that I did not tolerate things that were not right in my life, be that a physical "thing" or be it a relationship at work or even at home.

There is something about cancer that, once you have conquered it, makes you want to rid your life of things that are not working for you. Here are a few examples. Before cancer, if I was sorting through a box of items and came across something that was missing a piece, somehow broken, or non-functional in at least some minor way, I would say to myself, "Hmmm, this might be fixable or maybe I could use a part off of it for something else someday. I think I'll keep it." No more.

Right after cancer, when I would come across something broken, I wanted it out of my life. I would take a quick glance at something, notice that it was cracked or somehow not right, and straight into the trash it would go. I did not blink an eye. I did not hesitate one moment. Gone.

Why did this happen? Maybe it was a low tolerance for frustration. Maybe it was a sense that I was broken and once fixed, I wanted to minimize my interaction with things that were not just right. Whatever this is, it is a real emotion, a strong emotion, and it can be quite costly.

My friend who had leukemia, the one that called me prior to my surgery, had a similar feeling after his cancer treatments. He only would accept the best when purchasing anything. And I do mean anything. If he decided he needed new boots, they were Tony Lamas, custom made for his feet. If it was a musical instrument, it was a top of the line guitar or bass or maybe a new Yamaha concert grand piano, the largest they make. Nothing but the best would do and the price was no matter.

My first pangs of this problem came in the form of home fix-up. I am not a carpenter so I could not remodel the place but I had a strong sense of "something's got to be done" and a handy neighbor who was out of work.

My home was in the mountains and had not been updated since it was built in the 1960's. There was a bridge from the street over to the front door and it had become a bit too rickety to be safe. Armed with a fresh Home Depot credit card, I began with paint, continued with carpet, and had the neighbor do extensive reworking of the bridge.

Nothing in the house was left untouched by my hand. Kitchen cabinets got paint and decorative appliques. All tile floors were ripped up and redone. The bathroom was painted with new flooring to match. The office area where I would write was painted and reorganized.

The days went by and more and more tasks were accomplished. I was still weak from treatments so I would work awhile, rest a awhile, and then start in again. This methodology served me well. I could choose to give in to the weakness and let cancer win or work as much as I could, rest, and let the cancer lose.

When it was all said and done, I realized that now I do broken just fine. The house was much improved. I could feel comfortable there, and best of all I felt as refreshed as the place looked. There is a peace that comes over you when your surroundings are clean and in good order. Cancer amplifies the need for that peace. What you have to do is be careful about how much money you are willing to spend to create that peace.

Chapter Fourteen: Return to Nursing.

Thanks to short-term disability insurance (I highly recommend it), I had taken some time off from my stressful nursing work to focus on recovering from the cancer. While I enjoyed this time, I knew that the end was coming and that I would need to return to work. My registry service that I worked for was ready for me to come back and so one day, I got up the nerve to try working a shift.

My first shift back was at a hospital that I rarely worked. It was not my favorite but that is OK, I needed to get back to work. It was an adult ICU shift and I soon realized that I was not as strong as I thought I was. It was hard to drink enough water to keep my mouth moist and still abide by the rules of not keeping anything to drink at the nurses' station. I was tired, too tired to work as hard as I always had, and was definitely still burned out on nursing.

After that, I limited myself to pediatrics, as this usually does not require heavy lifting and always had been enjoyable to me. Soon, I switched to night shift as the drama and politics are much less than during the day. And finally, I got a call from the registry asking if I would like to do something really different. Would I be interested in filling-in as a nurse at a pediatric psychological services center,

8-5, Monday through Friday, for a couple of months? I jumped at the chance.

The work was not physically challenging, fit well with my skills, and gave me the break from bedside nursing that I desperately needed. Even more changes were in the works though. God plans these things and springs them on us quickly at times, slowly at other times. Some needed changes that I thought were slow in coming were about to burst on to the scene.

Chapter Fifteen: Who is Victoria and Why Would Someone Want to Kill Her?

Another one of those decisions that changes the entire course of our lives is whether or not to leave a marriage. Of all the decisions I have ever had to make, this has to be the most dramatic and life altering I have ever experienced.

After returning to work as a nurse and restarting my career as a drummer, I made that decision. The details of why I made that decision do not have to be aired here. There is no point in sharing those details in print. Take for granted the notion that given the same circumstances, you might make the same decision. If you have ever been divorced, just know that you did make the same decision, whatever your reasons and circumstances were. You probably would not want to see those details in print either.

If you have not been divorced, two thoughts come to mind. First, I hope you never need to divorce. It is painful, hurtful, tough on families, and expensive financially and emotionally. At no other time in life will treachery, envy, and hate threaten your sanity more than when you are in the throes of a divorce. Second, I hope you do not need to divorce and are putting off doing so. At no other time in life will treachery, envy, and hate threaten your sanity more than when you need to get a divorce and are trying to ignore that reality.

It was just prior to the separation of my marriage that I went on an audition for a heavy metal band that needed a drummer. Now I am not known at all as a heavy metal drummer. I do not listen to that style of music very often and had no experience with that type of drumming. But for an exercise, I decided to answer an ad placed on a local music store bulletin board for a band that called themselves "Kill Victoria."

After leaving a message at the number given, I got a call back from a nice voice that told me where online to find four demo songs. He arranged an audition time that would be just after a short trip to visit my sister in Iowa. I actually sat up late at night while at her home listening to the demo tunes over and over while writing out drum charts for the audition.

When I returned to California, I showed up at the address given and found a nice family home rumored to have been built sometime in the 1930's by a successful female country and western musician. In the garage, I found the three other members of Kill Victoria (two guitarists and a bass player) ready to see what this older drummer could do. I setup my drums, played hard, and got the gig.

Not that there was any money to be made, mind you. The other members of the band turned out to be ages 18, 19, and 20. Besides needing a drummer, I could be their chaperone when they played in venues that sold alcohol. But they wrote their own music, played their instruments very well, and had a passion for the music. I played with them for about a year and we recorded an album during that time. We played lots of shows and had a nice little fan-base that would come hear us play.

The house had a spare bedroom and I rented that for a short time after leaving my marriage. A palpable music vibe was always around that home and I attributed it to the ghost of the original owner. A grand piano graced the living room and it had been sold to the present homeowner along with the house. It was as if it was part of the house and meant to be there forever. It was fun to be living there but I was so much older that I really did not fit in well. It was not long before I made other arrangements and moved out.

And where did the name of the band come from? It originated from a very simple source. One of the band members had a girlfriend named Michelle. He called her one day and asked if they could go to the movies. "No, Victoria's coming over and we are going to the mall." Several times he called and asked her to go out and each time the reply was the same, "Victoria's coming over and we are going somewhere." Finally in frustration, he said, "Sometimes I could just kill Victoria." The other band members overheard this remark and the name Kill Victoria was decided upon.

One of the songs they wrote was entitled, "Still Not Dead." The first line of the lyric was, "Woke up this morning still not dead." I took that phrase and made it my motto for quite some time. I had survived cancer and I was still not dead.

I was involved in other music projects at the same time. I played in a much less threatening sounding group called "The Redlands East Valley Show Choir." Yes, I was a Glee drummer. Actually, this gig paid better than anything else I was doing musically. It was challenging as well. We would be called upon to play every style of music from jazz dance numbers to techno beats and even '60's oldies. The other musicians were friends I had worked with in various bands for many years.

I had turned down show choir at least twice before. That year was different though. I was determined to get out and play the drums as often as possible so when asked, I agreed to participate.

I mention show choir partially because I got to ride to one of the performances on a large bus. While going through my cancer treatments, one of the things I kept saying to myself when thinking about my life was, "I haven't been on the bus yet." What I meant by this was that I had played drums for many years, done lots of shows with various bands, but I had never been on a tour bus.

The first performance we booked involved riding to the venue on a tour bus. It of course was not the rock star version of a tour bus, with sleeping quarters, kitchen, and dual lounges. It was a standard people mover with upright seats but that did not matter to me. It was a bus and I was on the way to a music gig and that was enough. I had started my rock star status, if only in a mild-mannered way.

Bands come and bands go. After awhile, it was time for Kill Victoria to go. Show choir was done and a Janis Joplin tribute band that the show choir band had been working on was disbanding as well. I suddenly found myself once again wondering what was next.

My sister called when she heard the news and offered for me to stay with her in Iowa and switch my bedside nursing work over to a case management job she had seen in the local newspaper. Case management means that you are a nurse that does office work rather than direct patient care and I was ready for that. I packed a bag, left my drums and what few personal belongings I had after my divorce in a storage unit, and flew to Iowa.

Having cancer did not fix all my problems. It did point out to me that the problems were there and gave me the motivation to look to God for help and start trying to change things. They say in the song that when it comes to the Hotel California,

"You can checkout any time you want, but you can never leave." After a total of 24 years in that state, I paid my bill, grabbed my bags, and left the building. I checked out of the Hotel California. It was time to move on.

Chapter Sixteen: Welcome to Iowa

When you need help in life, do not be afraid to accept it when God brings it your way.

My sister and two of her three children, who now have children of their own, live in the same town in Iowa. When I arrived, I spent a lot of time resting. Change, even good change, comes through pain and I was hurting. I knew God did not want me to be in California anymore but I did not yet understand why.

The case management job interview went well and I began work shortly after arriving. The work was good and I tried to do well at it. My sister had connections with the local community college and soon I was teaching again too. The road to recovery is not just about getting over the physical problems. It is about becoming productive again and struggling to build a new future.

Sometimes that future doesn't look exactly like your original vision. Once I arrived in Iowa, I went about my usual manner of talking about my drumming life. Every day for two weeks straight, I would get the same response; "Hey, that's great that you play the drums. You don't happen to play bass do you?"

It didn't take long for me to wake up to the fact

that I should be learning the bass. I had often advised people to take up the bass when they asked me about being involved in music. Why? Every band needs a bass player and for the most part, no one wants to do it. Most people want to play guitar or keyboard, sing and be the star of the show. Others like the drums because it is an exciting, physical experience to play them. Not many people want to play the bass. But those that do, love it and are in high demand.

The drums and the bass make up the foundation of a band so in some ways, this would not be a terrible stretch for me. I had played bass a little over the years but had never studied it seriously. I visited the local Guitar Center, purchased a nice used Laguna bass guitar with case, and found a teacher.

When the instructor heard my story about being a life-long drummer, he said, "This will be easy for you. You already know how to read music and have some experience with music theory from your music degree. Mostly importantly, you already know how to be in a band."

I had never thought about it in quite that way, but there are certain skills that develop over time when play with other musicians in a band. You learn to pay attention to what the other players are doing so you can modify your part accordingly. You learn to watch for signals, some obvious, some non-verbal and not so obvious, about when we are starting, stopping, or modifying a song. You learn to synchronize your timing so that the music has that groove that makes people want to dance or buy your recordings. And most of all, you hopefully learn how to get along with other people. The instructor was right. I knew all that stuff. What I had to focus on was learning how to play the instrument.

Here's the surprising part. Within six weeks of beginning my bass lessons, I had an opportunity to substitute for the bass player in the contemporary Christian band at the church I had been attending. I received the materials, studied my parts, and showed up on Sunday morning for the early rehearsal. Singers will often want to change the key of a song from its original version but this didn't faze me at all due to my music theory background. We went over each tune, found our parts, and got ready for the service.

Once the service began, I remember focusing on my part and the other band members so much so that I did not realize how many people were in the congregation that morning. After the first couple of songs, I relaxed a bit and began to notice that I was playing in front of about four hundred people. This was amazing to me because in my club work with bands in the past, as anyone involved in music will tell you, you are lucky if you can get a hundred people to come out and see your band. Sure a lot of bands play before thousands of fans in theaters or arenas but ask almost any one of them and they will tell you they started out playing before small groups of family and friends. Here I am on bass, with only a few weeks of lessons, playing before a large, appreciative crowd. All I can think is that God is up to something.

Once in a while, God does you a favor. It seems like most of the time, God acts slowly and methodically. Sometimes, when you least expect it but need it the most, God comes at you like a bolt of lightening in the night sky.

I was lying in bed one morning about ten days before Christmas, praying from my heart. "I need something to go on, Lord. I need a boost." There was a drum clinic, that is what drummers call a training seminar, scheduled for that very night in Des Moines. I had been to the drum shop several times. It was owned by a good Christian couple and I enjoyed being there. No matter where you are in your drumming career, there is always something new to be learned so I decided to motivate myself and attend the clinic.

When I am talking with other drummers and I mention that I am a freelance writer for Modern Drummer magazine, it does not take long before I am deep in conversation about all things related to drumming. The instructor that night had an idea for a set of articles about working drummers, not the rock stars mind you, but the local drummers who teach kids all day, play clubs or churches the rest of the time, and hope for the occasional calls that come in to play with well-known artists.

When the clinic was over, the clinician invited me out for a bite to eat so we could discuss some article ideas he had for the magazine. After an evening of deep conversation about drums and drumming, he asked me, "What are you doing for the next couple of days?" I was off duty from my hospital job for several days so the next thing you know, he invites me to spend the weekend on a tour bus with a group from Iowa called "The Nadas."

The band had two gigs that weekend: Friday night in Omaha, Nebraska, and Saturday night in Sioux City, Iowa. I was allowed to travel with the band, sleep on the bus, and attend the gigs. As I was laying in my bunk the first night, I prayed. How could this not be a gift from God? I had lived my entire life wishing to travel on a tour bus and never feeling like I was in the right situation to go for that dream. Now here I was, on a bus once owned by a singer who goes by the name of "Meatloaf," traveling with a well-known band. You cannot put that together on your own.

Chapter Seventeen: Welcome to Arkansas

I swore I would never move back to Arkansas. I swore I would never get in a relationship with a girl from my hometown. Funny how some things happen despite all intent on your part to avoid them.

When I was in middle school and high school, I played in the school band but I also had a rock band on the side. We had a horn section and played a wide variety of music ranging from Chicago to Jimi Hendrix. We would play dances after football games, in the church basement for various functions, and really anywhere that would have us.

Each year, some members would graduate high school and disappear from the band and others would come into high school and join up. We had many great players in the band over the years and I developed lasting friendships with some of them.

One of those was the trombone player. He and I would contact each other occasionally through the years and much more in recent times. I mentioned to him one day that we should consider trying to have a reunion concert back in our hometown. He agreed and the groundwork was set for a life-changing experience that I did not see coming.

He found eleven guys that used to play in the

band and many of them could make the gig. A few substitute players had to be hired because three of the members had already passed away. Heart disease, mental illness, and HIV had taken a heavy toll on our group. A few rehearsals were scheduled and we were on our way.

What happened next, none of us could foresee. The concert was posted on Facebook and all of a sudden the event took on a life of its own. A multitude of old friends were sharing their plans to attend the concert. We had originally scheduled the community center but one friend said, "Too many of us are coming. You are going to have to find a larger place." That friend went to work on getting a larger venue and booked us into the high school auditorium. Another friend decided to arrange for food to be brought in for the band so we would not have to leave the venue between sound check and the performance.

The night of the show, 250 people attended. That might not sound like a lot to some people but this was in a small town of only 3000 residents. Some of the audience traveled from several states away just to hear us play. And we played well considering that the band had not been together in 35 years. We were shocked at the massive response.

We charged $5.00 admission with the intent to pay the substitute musicians and give the rest of the proceeds to the high school band program. We were pleased to give about a thousand dollars to the band department. In fact, one of the substitute musicians had such a good time that he gave the money back and made us promise to call him again if we ever did another show.

After the last song we announced that the band members would be down in front of the stage so old friends and family could come up and say hello. Then it began. For the next hour, we were literally mobbed by the crowd. People we had not seen in decades came up to greet us and tell us how much they enjoyed the music. We were truly rock stars that night.

One of those people was cancer survivor who knew my mother. She also has a daughter that is a cancer survivor just about my age. I was packing my drums and she came right up onto the stage and asked, "You gonna be in church tomorrow with your Daddy?"

"Yes Ma'am," I replied.

"We'll see you tomorrow then," she said and she was off. I knew her daughter when we were children growing up on adjacent farms and attended the same Sunday School. I had not seen her in a long time and had no idea that I was about to be seeing much more of her.

The next day after church, we all caught up in the parking lot and talked about our survival stories and plans they were making for a mission trip to Costa Rica.

We had been talking quite a while when my dad came up and mentioned that it was time to go to lunch. We all went to the same restaurant and sat together. Contact info was exchanged and the daughter and I started talking. I would not let myself think of anything more than a friendship for us at first, then something changed.

My next direct intervention from God came as an answer to another heartfelt prayer lifted up on my birthday. I had worked the night shift the evening before and slept most of the day. When I awoke, I had a sense that something more needed to be happening. Working in hospitals is stressful, drama-filled work that will sap every bit of life out of you that you let it get. I prayed earnestly, "There's got to be more to life than this. There has to be something that you want me to do more than this."

I had arranged to have five days off, starting with my birthday. I did not know what I would do when I arranged to have the time away but I knew that I needed to be gone. I had thought about going to Arkansas to visit family but something else kept coming to mind.

On the way down the highway toward Arkansas, I called the trombone player and arranged to have dinner with him and his fiancé. Then I called the daughter mentioned above and asked if she would like to go with me.

To make things even better, the trombone

player and fiancé were attending a Blood, Sweat, and Tears concert the next night. I had him get two extra tickets. We all enjoyed the show and after the concert, it was time to face up to what God had put before me. I had prayed for direction to what was next. Somehow that night, after the concert, in the parking lot of the Barnes and Noble, I realized where my life had been heading and agreed to go along. The Rock Star was no longer alone. There was something more to life and God had brought it to me.

Chapter Eighteen: You CAN Go Back Home Again

The upcoming marriage required a move, as she was finishing a career in government work and it did not make sense for her to forfeit that job when nursing work is easy to find. I called a hospital local to where she lived and basically told them, "I am a registered nurse with 20 years experience. What are you going to do with me?" We arranged an interview and another trip from Iowa to Arkansas was planned.

I interviewed for three positions, one of which I really thought I would enjoy. On the way back to Iowa, I prayed earnestly and boldly once again, saying, "God, I need some kind of sign. Is this move to Arkansas and the impending marriage the best thing that has ever happened or the craziest idea ever? I do not even know what kind of sign I need but I know I need one." Within five minutes, my cell phone rang. It was the manager over the job that I really wanted, making an offer that included a substantial salary increase over what I was currently making. I looked toward Heaven and understood that I had just had my sign handed to me. I soon found myself developing protocols and overseeing federal regulations in the Quality department of that local hospital. God provides and when that happens, it is good.

God did not stop with the job though. What I did not expect is that my music and writing careers would flourish. Arkansas is not known for its music scene other than a few tourist-oriented areas with folk or country music venues. What I came to understand relates to the phrase, "Bloom where you are planted."

One of the problems with trying to be a professional drummer in the Los Angeles area is that there are a lot of drummers living there. A whole lot. And they are good too. Trained in the latest styles and techniques, if an audition comes around you can safely expect that 100 great drummers will show up. That makes the competition for work very tough.

In Arkansas, the numbers are very different. If the local community theater is putting on a show, they will be lucky if they can find anyone to play the drums, much less someone good. Churches all over the place need musicians to cover services and since I could play a little bass too, I could work as much as I wanted. The trombone player I have been talking about is involved in so many music projects, he has a rehearsal or a performance almost every night of the week. Try that in LA.

And the writing career? I got more assignments after the move than I had done in years. The Internet is the great leveler of all things. If you have any kind of internet connection, living in a rural state does not mean that you are not plugged in to the latest, greatest whatever thing and can continue to research and submit your writing work the same as if you were in downtown Los Angeles or New York. No difference at all, other than Arkansas is much more peaceful and affordable. Talk about your winning combination.

And access to rock stars? Much better in the rural South. How can that be, you ask? Set up your interview for bands visiting Tunica, Mississippi. It is a small gambling area along the Mississippi River just south of Memphis, Tennessee. When you try to arrange an interview in Los Angeles, the drummer is always busy with the record company reps, the drum manufacturer he is endorsing, or any number of other distractions that are begging for his or her attention. In Tunica, there is literally nothing to do. I discovered this sitting on a tour bus interviewing the drummer for Train for an hour with no interruptions, no distractions, and no rush on his part to get me out the door. Unbelievably easy to schedule and do. Amazing.

And of course, there I was on a tour bus again, this time with the new wife along. How is all this happening? There God goes again is really the only answer I could come up with.

Chapter Nineteen: The Nurse Becomes a Rock Star

When you are five years out from cancer treatment, and the cancer has not returned, you get to use the other "C" word, "cured." Actually, I do not use that word very often. You see, I understand that "cured" is a precarious condition. I did not expect the first bout with cancer and I do not expect another but having been a nurse for almost all of my adult life, I know it can and does happen. Even so, I wake each morning confident that today will not be the day it returns. I have survived well, made the changes that were begging to be made, and basically started living all over again. There was only one problem remaining. I was not a rock star yet.

My wife calls me "Rock Star Rick" and sure, I feel like one when she says that, but I had never performed on a big arena stage to a large crowd of fans. Maybe it is a bit self-indulgent to think that is a desirable thing to do. I have been in the audience at large concerts often enough to know that it is a thing that happens out there in the world. As much as I understand that humbleness is a virtue, I still dreamed of finding myself on a large stage, with professionally run lights and sound, playing my heart out on the drums while I still could.

Time for another intervention from God. Sometimes, God not only surprises you when you least expect it, it is done in a roundabout way you would never imagine in a million years.

A friend had recruited my wife to become a representative for a skin care company called Rodan and Fields. I was skeptical at first but had no reason not to go along so I started working the business with her. Not long after that, she decided to go to the annual company convention in Dallas, Texas. "Sure, I'll go too," I told her when she asked.

A little time goes by and I receive an e-mail asking people associated with the company who have talent to sign up for a show to be held on Saturday night during the convention. I was reluctant to respond, thinking, "No one is going to want to see someone up on stage banging on the drums by themselves." At the urging of my spouse, I let her film a short video of me to meet the submission requirements and sent it off to the corporate offices.

The deadline for selection notification passed and I had not heard anything back from my entry so I resigned myself to the rejection and did not think anything more of it. The next thing you know, an e-mail arrives a few days after Christmas, my favorite holiday remember, and I have been invited to be part of the show.

A few more days go by before I get a call from the corporate office. The video of me playing drums had made the rounds and they had an idea. They asked if I would agree to allow some of the office workers who were also musicians to play along with me. They would take care of rewriting the lyrics of a popular song to match a product release that was planned for the convention.

The video I sent was of me playing on a spare drum set that I had purchased used for $150 and recovered in zebra print using thick wrapping paper. The recovering job was done so the kit would match some furnishings in a jungle-themed living room. This meant the kit blended into the decor enough that it could be left set up all the time. The office workers thought it would be cool if the guitar player dressed up in zebra print pants to match the kit.

"What song?" I asked. "Pour Some Sugar on Me by Def Leopard" was the response. OK, I thought. What could it hurt? That would be a good crowd participation song and they said I could take a solo at the beginning of the tune and again in the middle. That is cool and way more latitude than you get as a drummer in most bands. I agreed and the rehearsal and performance times were set.

Then came the kicker. "By the way Rick, the performance will be held in the arena at the Dallas Convention Center in front of an estimated audience of 5000."

Sometimes you prayerfully wait for something for years and you feel like nothing is happening toward your desire. Then all of a sudden comes the final piece that signals the culmination of countless small pieces of a large puzzle that was years in the making. Your dream, or rather God's version of it, which will do quite nicely thank you, is at hand. It happens when you least expect it, in ways that you cannot imagine. And it is good.

Never mind the fact that I would be playing on the cheapest drum kit I own. The sound of the kit was good or I never would have purchased it. I would supplement the zebra colored drums with pro-level gear from my life-long collection, including a snare drum I built on my own and stick bag given to me by my sister.

I am a perfectionist when it comes to good tuning. No matter how well you play, if the drums sound bad, you sound bad. I play the best I can play every time I sit down behind the kit and I bring the best sounding gear possible. There is never a good reason to do anything less. During rehearsal, the sound tech even commented on what great tone the kit had and how well I had it tuned.

The night of the performance came. It was just the one song, part of a long show with several speeches and a few other music performances. When they announced my name, I ran out on stage, sat down behind the drums, and immediately began to play.

I have done many solos over the years so I was used to that part of it. I grew up watching the great Buddy Rich blast through drum-oriented tunes with a smile on his face that relayed his passion for the instrument. I have shared that passion all my life. I marched in my first parade at age 11. I have hauled drums in and out of clubs, churches, and outdoor park stages since I was 13 years old. And now, here I was. Playing in an arena to thousands.

But I really did not see them. The lights on stage are such that you can see the first few rows of the audience but other than that, the seating area is fairly dark. The other musicians came out on stage at the appropriate moment and the tune began. My second solo came and went. We wrapped up the last verse and chorus, gave a quick wave to the crowd, and off stage we went.

I caught up with the lead guitar player in the dressing room. "How do you think it went?"

He looked me straight in the eye and said, "Rick, didn't you see the audience. We had them on their feet. They loved it."

"No," I replied, "I didn't see them." I had been so focused on the solos and playing the groove, that is what drummers call the rhythm pattern of a song, that I did not see how the audience responded.

That is OK though. I understand that playing music is not about getting gratification for myself. It is about fulfilling a destiny that I trust was formed for me before I was born. God sets the doors and the forks in the road in front of us and we have freedom of choice about some of the paths we travel in life but I truly believe that each decision that we make has consequences, good or bad, that shape the remainder of our lives after that. Post cancer, I watched closely and followed God's lead. By doing so, I rebuilt a life that included tour buses, arena-sized audiences, and a wonderful marriage. To say it does not get any better than that would be an understatement but oh so true.

After the Dallas show, we were taken back to the hotel to an after-party for convention attendees. Everywhere I went that night, audience members were coming up to me and telling me how much they enjoyed my part of the show. I could not walk down the hall to my room without someone coming up all smiles and complimenting me on my performance. I was truly a rock star that night.

I generally do not let myself feel too good about anything. I think I have to work all the time in order to be better at whatever it is I am doing. Hospital work, music, writing, family life; I work hard at all of these. I do not rest on my laurels, that is for sure. I do not let myself get over-confident. And I do not let myself feel good about things for fear that complacency will set in and I will lose everything I have gained.

Ask my wife and she will tell you that once in a while after a successful event of some kind, I will say, "I am going to let myself feel good about this for five minutes." That night, after my first arena show, I let myself feel good about it for five minutes. Those were five really great minutes.

The road to becoming a rock star is a road full of potholes, paved with gravel, with large ditches on both sides. I had been towed out of one of the ditches with my cancer episode. That evening, the bumpy road I had traveled all my life felt a little smoother.

Chapter Twenty: Oh, But God's Not Done

Turns out I'm not the only one with a dream in this marriage. After much contemplation, and a year of scholarship searching and application submission, my wife is ready to answer the call to become a minister by attending seminary. We up and move to Kansas City as part of this process and on the way to our new place of residence, my wife says, "You've wanted to be a full-time musician all your life. Make that happen."

The Kansas City area has a vibrant music scene that is mostly unknown to the rest of the world. Upon arriving in town, it took all of four hours for me to be approached by someone who needed a replacement drummer in his band for the summer. I also started attending one of the local jam sessions for jazz musicians and using the network marketing skills I had learned from the skincare business to try and make my full-time musician vision into reality. It worked, but with a bit of a twist.

I quickly found that Kansas City had a lot of competent drummers available. Even so, I got a call to fill in for a drummer on a 1920-30's style jazz one-nighter at a local coffee shop. The coronet player who hired me cornered me after the last set. ""I have a regular drummer who just couldn't be here tonight but I heard you talking about also playing bass. I really need a permanent bass player."

I explained to him that I had taken a few lessons in Iowa and substituted at church but really did not know how to play jazz bass. "What's your point?" he responded. I explained again that I really did not know jazz bass. His response was, "You don't understand. I need a bass player. Rehearsal is Sunday night at 6pm. Be there."

Here was one of those moments in life where you either turn and walk away from opportunity or you seize it and run with it. I looked at this guy and said, "OK. If you will be nice to me the first few rehearsals until I can get this walking bass line thing figured out, I'll be there." He agree and for the next two and half years, I had a weekly jazz brunch gig at a great club with a long list of permanent and guest musicians that are some of Kansas City's finest.

Other bass gigs starting coming in quickly. I soon found myself in two Pink Floyd tribute band projects, a Stevie Ray Vaughn tribute band, a jazz-reggae band, and a couple of rock music projects too. In each case, I was learning so much and growing as a musician. The skills I learned on bass made me a much better drummer as well, since my understanding of various musical styles was expanding and my overall experience was increasing.

God saw to it that I still gained experience on the drums too. I auditioned for, and was accepted into, a spot playing drums for a contemporary Christian service at The United Methodist Church of the Resurrection. This is the largest church in the United States that is of a major denomination. A few independent churches are larger but as far as Baptist, Methodist, Presbyterian, etc., this is the largest church as its membership at that time was about 24,000. On any given Sunday, the service I played for would number about 1500 or more in attendance at the church and another 2,000-3,000 or more online.

This was a great opportunity because the level of musicianship there is amazing and the complexity of the music was challenging. What started for me as a six or seven piece worship band grew into a situation that occasionally used a 14-piece studio orchestra and a choir of about 30 voices. Think about what The Moody Blues would sound like if they played contemporary Christian music and this was it.

On Christmas Eve of 2013, I had been asked to play two of the many Christmas Eve services held at Church of the Resurrection. Our music team opened with "Christmas Eve/Sarajevo 12/24" by The Trans Siberian Orchestra, one of the most powerful and dynamic Christmas instrumentals ever written in my humble opinion. For the remaining tunes, I shared the drum kit with the other drummer on our team so that we all could be involved that day. I took to the tympani or other percussion when not on the kit.

The blessing of this day was not only the music and the chance to serve God but also the number of people in attendance. At each service, the sanctuary was filled to its capacity of 3000 with 500 more out in the lobby. Those 500 would come into the sanctuary for the candle lighting portion of the service near the end, thus making it so that we were playing in front of 3500 people at each service. I had never played to 7000 people in a day before but here, just six years out from the very worst days of my cancer episode, I was living one of my best days.

After the service, I went out to my car in the cold, snowy parking lot, got inside, and sat there for a few minutes, not moving at all. I was praying. I prayed earnestly and boldly, "God, how did you do that? How did we go from having cancer to playing the drums in front of 7000 people at the largest Methodist church in the country?"

You see, the part I haven't written about yet is my prayer upon first learning that I had cancer. My greatest worry was not that I might die but that I would have to face God without having fully developed and used my talent for playing music. I truly believe talent comes from above and somehow I knew that God wasn't done with me yet. I felt that I had followed God's lead to become a nurse and to spend my life taking care of those around me, both at the hospitals were I worked and at home, but I felt unresolved about music and its role in my life. I felt deep down that I should be doing more with music and somehow knew that God felt that way too.

I prayed about it, saying, "Lord, I feel that you are not done with me. Let's get through this cancer episode and get on to the future that you have in store for me. I like the new contemporary Christian music. Maybe you have a spot for me where I can serve you and use my music talent to the fullest." Six years later there I sat, in the parking lot of a church I had never heard of, in a town I never thought I'd live in, married to a person studying to be a minister, and playing drums in front of 7000 people and bass recently in front of hundreds more.

In my mind, I could hear God's answer. "We did it one small step at a time." And that truly is how it happened. I had to get through the cancer treatments, leave California, study bass in Iowa, marry a childhood friend in Arkansas, move to Kansas City, and so on. Each small step in the process was important in its own way. Six years of small steps, taken one day at a time, one step at a time. Not so long really but so very, very far.

Chapter Twenty-One: We Are All Rock Stars

So I had cancer and I became a rock star.

The point I have been leading up to with this book is that in truth, we are all rock stars. We all have a song to sing; something we want to say in life. We all have an instrument that we play well. It may be a computer, a vacuum cleaner, or a stethoscope but it is our instrument and we like to play it.

We all have a favorite venue. Maybe it is the living room, or the boardroom, but we can't wait to play there again.

We all have a fan base. People who want to be near us, know more about us, or emulate us are all around. They may be friends from work or church or maybe our children or grandchildren. No matter. They are loyal fans who love the song we sing with our instrument.

And we all have things in our lives that we hope the tabloid magazines never print. Nobody's perfect but never forget that our fans think we are.

So grab your instrument, practice your song, sign-up to play your favorite venue, and take your act on the road. Your fans are depending on you. Don't let it take cancer to bring out your inner rock star.

The next time you need a change in your life, look in the mirror. Gaze into your own eyes. There is a light inside them; a sparkle that has always been there. Look for it when you are feeling your worst and let it be the beacon that brings you back to strength, life, and love. That light will never go out. It is your soul. And I believe your soul lives forever.

Even so, you only really ever have "the now." Forgive yourself of any wasted time in the past, keep your eyes toward the future and plan for better times as much as Fate will permit, but live, everyday, in the now. Work today to make your "now" what you want it to be. You do your part and God will do God's part. Working together with Fate, instead of fighting against it, will create a better "now" than you could ever imagine.

After all, I was a nurse. I had cancer. Now I'm a rock star.

Epilogue: Five Years Out and Counting

My surgeon told me that most people who have a recurrence of throat cancer do so within two years. He also said if you get to five years out without problems, your chance of recurrence is very low. I am happy to say that I made it to five years out, and beyond, and life is good. I keep my follow-up visits to the doctor and exercise regularly. The changes that I made have taken me places I never thought I would go. When you spend your life following God, that is what happens.

Faith is believing in something you cannot see or prove. I have a strong faith in God. I cannot prove scientifically to you that God has led me to the place and situation I am in today but I can say that I arrived here by listening to that still, small voice in the back of my head, the thought behind the thought, that seemed to be guiding me through it all. I know for sure where I would be if I had not listened to that voice. Still lost. You see, I once was lost, as the song says, but now am found. Was blind to the problems of life and was dying of cancer, but now I see.

Appendix: Nurse Rick's Tips and Tricks for Surviving Head and Neck Cancer

First and foremost, if you have been diagnosed with cancer you are about to go through an experience that will save your life and change your life at the same time. It will not be easy but it won't be that hard considering the alternative.

From day one, you are going to find out who your friends are. Some will surprise you and some will disappoint you. Let those that disappoint you go. You don't need them anyway. Embrace those that surprise you and accept their support.

Everyone has heard of cancer. Not many people know what it is. You learned in high school biology class that your cells divide and make new cells all the time. The new cells are exactly like the old cells, hopefully. If something happens, and the new cells are not the same, problems can occur.

Sometimes the new cell is a different type of cell. We've had surgeons open up a patient and find a tooth where a tooth should not be. This doesn't really hurt anything and is typically called a benign tumor. Sometimes the new cell is a type that spreads the mistake around and this is known as a malignant tumor.

Yes, cancer is more complicated than what I've just said but really, this is all you need to know about it. You drive your car around town everyday and you don't understand all the thermodynamics of internal combustion engines do you? Don't worry about the cancer or how you got it. Worry about how you are going to get rid of it.

If you have a head/neck cancer, like mine was, it may be squamous cell cancer. This is a type of skin cancer. Skin lines your throat and sinuses. It is also likely that you didn't know you had this cancer until it spread to the lymph nodes in your neck and caused a lump. Usually, spreading to the lymph nodes is not what you want since it means the cancer could be on its way to other parts of the body through the lymph system.

With squamous cell cancer, even if it has spread to nearby lymph nodes, it tends to sit there and not move around the body like other cancers. Head/neck cancers are often found when they spread to the lymph nodes because it is difficult to detect yourself that you have a cancer growing in your throat. Again, don't worry about this. This is just how it is.

There are three ways to get rid of cancer: surgery, radiation, and chemotherapy. Holistic health practitioners will tell you some other methods. I won't tell you they are wrong. Maybe they are right. I got rid of mine with surgery, radiation, and chemotherapy. Each person with cancer has to choose their own treatment from what is available.

If possible, your doctor will have you undergo surgery to remove the cancerous tissues. Get some rest before the surgery. You may be nervous about the procedure but trust that the surgeon has done a lot of surgeries before and will do well with yours. Remember, surgeons do surgery all the time. He or she knows what they are doing or they wouldn't touch you. Any lawyer will be glad to tell you why.

Surgeons don't mind passing difficult patients off to a more experienced colleague. If you get comfortable with your doctor and then they want to refer you to someone else, trust that the new doc is the one for the job even if you don't like them personally as well as the first doc. You are not trying to make new friends here. You are trying to survive.

After surgery, rest. Remember all those times when you wished you could take a nap in the afternoon and were just too busy? Now you are not too busy. In fact, a nap should be the first thing on your priority list.

And all those friends and family members that call you with some new daily drama episode? Tell them you'll get back to them next year. Now is the time to take care of yourself, not everyone else.

The next step after surgery may be radiation. This is where you lie on a table in a room with a big machine that looks like some kind of scanner device in a science fiction movie. Actually, it is. It sends out radio waves at your body that are focused on the area of your cancer. It moves around and sends the beams at you from different directions. This takes about 10 minutes for most cancers. Head and neck areas are more difficult and they require two sessions back to back thus making the treatment just over 20 minutes.

Before your first treatment, go to the health food store and buy some pure aloe vera gel. It has to be pure; no perfumes. After each radiation treatment, when you get up from the table, put this on your face and neck. Put this stuff on and don't care how it looks. It won't look that bad anyway. This will keep your face from drying out and may help keep your skin from breaking down.

One day after treatments, you will put on the aloe gel and it will feel like it dried your skin rather than helped it. Go now to the radiation oncologist and get a prescription for Biafine cream. Use it like you did the aloe from then until the end of treatments. The goal here is to prevent skin breakdown. Do what you have to do.

You are going to look like you are sunburned. Buy yourself some new clothes. Get an orange sweatshirt or t-shirt, depending on the season. The orange color will keep you from looking so red when you go out in public.

Speaking of the public, avoid crowds and large stores while you are in treatment for cancer. Your immune system will be on break for a while. Don't put your self at risk for viruses and bacteria that are going around.

When you have head/neck radiation, you have to be locked to the table with a mask that looks like Jason from the Friday the 13th movie series. This is so you don't move your head thus allowing the radiation beam to always hit the same area. This can be difficult if you are claustrophobic.

My suggestion for everyone is to play some music during the treatment. Don't play your favorite songs. You don't want to start associating them with the treatment. Instead, put on some loud alternative rock or wild jazz and crank it up to about 100 decibels. This will keep you distracted and the time will pass more quickly. My radiation tech suggested this and it worked well. Take your own boom box if they don't have one. You won't be disturbing anyone. There's no one in the radiation room but you and the walls are lead-lined. Crank it up everyday.

Your throat is about to be sore. This will feel like the worst sore throat you've ever had. The doctor will prescribe a mixture of nystatin and lidocaine that you can gargle and swallow. Do it. Do it every four hours. Especially do it before you eat. I did this every four hours for three months.

After radiation, while you are walking to your car, open your mouth wide and say "ahhhhhh" and go from a medium pitch to a low pitch. This will stretch your throat. Then look far to the left and far to the right. This is range of motion for your neck. You don't want to lose any range of motion and you will if you don't stretch it out left and right everyday. Keep doing this for many years after the treatments since scar tissue develops over time.

After all this, you will be at the car. Head over to a drive-in and get something to eat. This will exercise the muscles necessary for swallowing. You don't want to lose function there and many people do.

What you won't be able to avoid is that your taste buds and saliva glands are going to be changed by the radiation. Many foods and fluids won't taste the same but some will. Experiment until you find things to eat and drink that taste good to you. The selections will vary from person to person. Just eat and drink and don't worry about your cholesterol right now. Eat to live and to maintain your weight.

Immediately stop smoking and drinking alcohol. Period. Your liver is going to be busy enough with the work it has to do to process the toxins in your treatments. Beside, you knew you needed to do this anyway, right? Now you have to. It might be tough at first but remember, the cancer is going to change your life for the better. This might just be one way it does that.

You will feel more tired as the radiation treatments continue. If you need someone to drive you to treatments, don't be shy about asking. I drove myself right up to the end but it was my daily project to do so and was all I did during the final few treatments.

The best advice my surgeon gave me was, "Listen to your body." If you are tired, nap. If you are hungry, eat. If you aren't making much urine, drink even if you aren't thirsty. You body is telling you it is thirsty in a different way. Bored? Find something to do. Listen to your body. It won't lie to you about what it needs.

Chemotherapy is a fancy word for chemical therapy. Called chemo for short, it involves poisoning you. Yes, I said it. You are about to be poisoned. The idea behind this treatment is to make every cell in your body sick. The weak cancerous ones will die and the others will survive and return to health.

The problem side effect most people have with chemo is nausea and vomiting. The problem here, besides the discomfort, is that you are losing fluids at a time when it may be difficult for you to drink because of the sore throat issues with the radiation. The nurses and doctors will give you something to take to counteract the nausea. Take it. It will be an anti-nausea drug and a steroid that will act as an anti-inflammatory. You will take these the day you receive chemo and for a few days after-wards.

My suggestion is to ask the doctor to let you also take these meds for three days ahead of the chemo dose. I found that this kept me from having the severe nausea and vomiting that I had with the first dose of chemo. The meds are given in small doses anyway so a few extra days will not present a problem and in fact could save you much of the agony of chemo-related nausea.

Remember that nausea is a hydration problem. If you feel nauseated, drink fluids. Sounds like the opposite advice you would usually hear but it works. If you notice that you aren't urinating as often as you usually would, you are getting dehydrated. Drink. If this isn't enough, go to the chemo nurses and ask them to give you a liter of normal saline through an IV. How much better you will feel is worth the needle stick.

Hair loss is another side effect of chemo. Try this:

don't wash your hair on the day of your chemo treatment and for two or three days after that. When you wash your hair, you pull on it and this can help pull it out. Just leave it alone. There is no beauty contest going on at the chemo department.

Radiation and chemotherapy can lower your appetite. If you find that you don't want to eat, have the doctor prescribe Megace. This medication is actually a man-made version of a female hormone involved in pregnancy. The med will increase your appetite sufficiently but you may find yourself crying over a romantic movie or an old song you hear on the radio. Don't ask me how I know.

At the other end, chemotherapy will either give you diarrhea or constipation. Treat each one accordingly because both will cause you further problems that you can avoid if you will just deal with the problem up front. Again, you doctor can prescribe something that will help.

Another prescription that will help is Prozac. When this drug first came on the market, it gained some negative publicity due to several cases of suicide. The problem was that it worked so well, people that were severely depressed and barely functioning in life began to feel well enough to do themselves in. You are likely not that depressed but how could you have cancer and not get depressed about it? It is OK to be upset about this! Take some Prozac, decide to live, and go for it.

Now that you are feeling "up" from the Prozac, laugh. Put on a cartoon DVD from your childhood or a favorite old comedy show. Laugh till it hurts. Think back about your childhood or young adulthood when you felt well. Get in touch with that feeling and hold on to it for dear life. Literally.

Next, find a project. Mine was converting old family slides to digital files so they wouldn't continue to deteriorate. The project does not need to be expensive. The attachment for the digital camera was only a few dollars. I converted 1,200 slides during my treatments. I posted them on-line for family across the country to see. You wouldn't believe the joy this brought to others and to me. Some of the pictures had not been seen in many decades. Find a project that makes a difference in your life and in the lives of your family and/or friends and get started on it.

Also important is laughter and good feelings. Think back about a television show that you enjoyed as a child or maybe a series of movies you liked. Buy the series on DVD and watch a few episodes each day. Laugh or feel good while watching this. It takes you back in your mind to a time when you were healthy and felt better. This will help you stay anchored to good feelings that will help you through your treatments.

Remember earlier when I said you were going

to become a different person? Allow your self to imagine working in a different job, living in a different area, or doing something that you have always wanted to do. Now is the time to make the changes in life that you have always wanted to make. There is no sane reason not to.

Made in the USA
Columbia, SC
19 November 2024

47011898R00088